PRAISE FOR ADRENALINE NATION

"As the former vice president for human resources at several world renowned companies, I know what works and what doesn't in the employee benefits arena. Peter McCarthy's *Adrenaline Nation* addresses a topic that is rarely discussed but has significant impact on the productivity of the employee and the ultimate results of the business. This book will help countless employees, and their companies, implement innovative, effective solutions in the workplace that will directly impact the bottom line and, equally important, the health of the workforce for the better. This book is a must-have for everyone who works in Corporate America."
– **Glenna Hecht, President, Humanistic Consulting, LLC**

"Peter McCarthy, TN is a dynamic leader, a brilliant and practiced naturopath, and a passionate spokesman for the cause of natural health. With *Adrenaline Nation*, he hits the bull's eye on the subject of chronic stress! I see its effects daily in my practice with my own clients. His in-depth prescriptions for both individuals and businesses will revolutionize the way we all think about stress. *Adrenaline Nation* is destined to be a bible for those who want to know more about the subject of stress in the workplace."
– **Gary Avignon, Licensed Psychotherapist, Author,** *Weight Wizardry 101: Introduction to the Psychology of Successful Weight Control;* **www. mindfulweigh.com**

"Once in each generation true genius may come, more often than not, only once or twice in a century. *Adrenaline Nation*, the new ground breaking text from Peter McCarthy, represents true genius and remarkable insights. This refreshingly powerful, compelling work should be at the very core of everyone's thinking, from citizen families to health care providers, business leaders and most especially legislators at local, state and federal levels. Practical, penetrating, and provocative are his solutions to change this complex, confusing and misunderstood issue which affects each of us in direct and very personal ways. I cannot recommend this book highly enough, and consider it a treasured addition in my reference library. You will, too."
– James R. Bowman, MD, ND, DNHC, DCP, FAAIM, Founder and Clinical Director, Alternative Health Concepts, LLC

"As an expert in business productivity, I applaud *Adrenaline Nation's* comprehensive approach to striking the correct balance between employee productivity and well-being. This book offers a winning strategy for employees and businesses alike."
– Dave Crenshaw, Author, *Invaluable: The Secret to Becoming Irreplaceable*

"I've walked the halls of the capitol in Austin with Peter McCarthy, and know first hand his passion and commitment for natural health advocacy. *Adrenaline Nation* showcases his extensive background in all aspects of human health. Not just the mind, but the body, spirit and how stress influences your state of being. This book is a must read for anyone that feels the stressful effects of living in the 21st century!"
– Keith Klein, Certified Clinical Nutritionist; Owner, Institute of Eating Management and Relapse Prevention Center; Author, *Weight Control for A Young America, Get Lean, Beyond Diet*

"*Adrenaline Nation* is a must read for every thinking American. Author Peter McCarthy tackles the many sacred health care cows nobody else has the courage to discuss, and skillfully explains how we can think boldly in new directions to create real change."
– **Elissa Meininger, Founder, Health Freedom Action Network; Former Vice President, *Friends of Freedom International*; Columnist, *News With Views*; Health Policy Analyst, *Super Health*, Fox Sports Radio 1340 AM, Oklahoma City**

"When Peter McCarthy co-wrote a health care policy paper for use by the Obama administration, he was endorsed by thousands of health advocates and health freedom organizations across the country and established himself as a major policy contributor in our nation's health care debate. Now, with *Adrenaline Nation*, he has combined that policy expertise with his business management skills to help the US business community fashion practical, effective solutions for one of its most intractable problems: combating the effects of chronic employee stress. *Adrenaline Nation* is a must-read for every business leader!"
– **Diane Miller, JD, Director of Law and Public Policy, National Health Freedom Coalition**

"A fascinating look at the whole picture of stress and how it affects our health. *Adrenaline Nation* presents an amazing amount of information, covering the wide spectrum of stress factors, but also showing how they work together in a holistic manner. Mainstream medicine virtually ignores almost all of these factors even though stress is a significant source of disease and illness. I can testify from personal experience that most of us don't appreciate what stress can do to our health until it's too late. Great job!"
– **Alan Smith, Author, *UnBreak Your Health***

"Peter McCarthy has emerged as a powerful national voice for health reform and holistic health care. In *Adrenaline Nation*, Peter identifies positive, innovative solutions which will restore health in the American business community and drastically lower costs in the long run."

– Mary Zennett, MD, MBA, Author, *Health For US All: The Transformation of US Health Care*; Director, Medical Design and Services, Wings of a Dream Foundation

"Peter McCarthy's *Adrenaline Nation* offers incisive analysis and easy-to-understand prescriptions for solving the problem of chronic stress in the corporate workplace. *Adrenaline Nation* will be a corporate reference bible for years to come!"

– Jill Lublin, International speaker and author of the national bestselling books, *Networking Magic, Guerrilla Publicity*, and *Get Noticed, Get Referrals*.

"*Adrenaline Nation* is brilliant! Peter McCarthy is on the cutting edge of how to identify and achieve a stress free life. His resolutions are powerful and offer a win-win for all parties involved that can literally change the world. It's thought provoking, life improving and best I've ever read!"

- Wendy Ida, Master Fitness Trainer & Columnist, Author *Take Back Your Life*

"*Adrenaline Nation* brings to light the largely unknown factors which impact our body's stress response. Peter McCarthy's clear and incisive explanations leave no doubt that our society has imposed an unsustainable stress load on all of us. He offers us a way out."

- Cindy Griffin, DSH-P, Founder, Homeopathy Center of Houston

Adrenaline Nation

Chronic Stress is Ruining Our Health and Bankrupting Our Economy

Peter M. McCarthy

Adrenaline Nation

Peter M. McCarthy

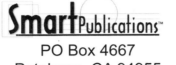

PO Box 4667
Petaluma, CA 94955
www.smart-publications.com

Published in the United States of America

First Edition, 2012

Library of Congress Control Number: 2011943445

ISBN: 1-890572-23-3   978-1-8905722-3-5

Warning—Disclaimer

Smart Publications™ has designed this book to provide information in regard to the subject matter covered. It is sold with the understanding that the publisher and the author are not liable for the misconception or misuse of the information provided. Every effort has been to make this book as complete and as accurate as possible. The purpose of this book is to educate and entertain. The author and Smart Publications™ shall have neither liability nor responsibility to any person or entity with respect to any loss, damage caused, or alleged to have been caused, directly or indirectly, by the information contained in this book.

"Smart Publications" is a trademark of Morgenthaler Family Limited Partnership, a Nevada Limited partnership.

About the Author

Peter M. McCarthy, TN, a traditional naturopath, is a well-respected and sought after professional in the field known as complementary and alternative medicine (CAM). He is CEO of AHI Productions, a media company which is the creator of NHN TV, the planet's first television network devoted to natural health and green living news, education, and entertainment.

He earned a Doctorate in Traditional Naturopathy from Trinity College of Natural Health in 2003, and was nationally board certified in 2005. He is a past member of the Advisory Committee of the American Naturopathic Certification Board; President of the Texas Complementary and Alternative Medical Association; and Chair of the Texas Health Freedom Coalition, the nation's largest state level grass roots natural health advocacy network, with over 50,000 members.

He graduated from the US Air Force Academy in 1972 with a BS in Engineering Mechanics and an Air Force commission as a second lieutenant. A 20 year military veteran, he earned an MA in Management and Supervision from Central Michigan University while on active duty.

He became a Captain/First Officer for Southwest Airlines in mid-1993 and served there until his retirement in mid-2009. It was during this time that his interest in naturopathy developed as he began to see the impact of stressors on the health of those around him, both in his professional and his personal life.

Peter and his wife Nancy live in Austin, TX. Together they have three grown children.

DEDICATION

To Margie R.
Thank you for your inspiration and courage.
I kept my promise.

To the Natural Health Practitioner and
Advocate Communities.
Thank you for your perseverance and dedication to true
health and individual freedom in the face
of overwhelming odds.
We will prevail.

To my wife, Nancy.
Without you, I could not.

ACKNOWLEDGMENTS

Any author who has the good fortune to have a book published, especially in the current environment, owes that good fortune to a team of people who were steadfast in support of the creative process, from start to finish.

Many, many thanks to John Morgenthaler, Smart Publications publisher and fellow health freedom advocate, who saw the vision of what *Adrenaline Nation* was trying to accomplish and threw his wholehearted support behind bringing its message to the world.

Likewise, profound thanks to my editor, Cristina Baggese, who made what otherwise could have been a trying process, an absolute pleasure. Would that all of you authors out there could have an editor like mine!

My wonderful, persistent and supportive agent, John Willig of Literary Services, Inc., has been an unfailing coach, adviser and fan of *Adrenaline Nation* since its inception. Thanks, John, for holding my feet to the fire!

Randy Peyser, founder of Author One Stop, has provided sage advice every step of the way, and introduced me to John Willig. Thank you Randy!

Unbeknownst to most, *Adrenaline Nation* was a four year project, which began with me learning to transform my writing style from the magazine article format to what you now hold in your hands. This could not have occurred without the steadfast support, encouragement and tutelage of my friend and advocate, Philippa

Burgess of Creative Convergence. Her patience, as well as her willingness to also hold my feet to the fire, were indispensable elements in the success of this book.

Thanks to my editorial readers, Robin Sherwood and Becky Howell, ND, RPh, for their encouragement, support and editorial advice.

Thanks also to the three men who, unbeknownst to them, helped start me on this path: Dr. Rob Cass, ND, naturopathic physician and founder of the Energetix Corporation; Dr. I. Michael Borkin, NMD, whose groundbreaking endocrine research expanded my horizons and helped me think differently about stress; and Dr. Datis Kharrazian, DC, whose genius has helped propel the need for chronic stress management to the forefront of public consciousness.

Thanks to my business partner and friend, Radhia Gleis, CCN, MEd, PhD, who offered steadfast encouragement and enthusiasm every step of the way.

Thanks to my success coach, Catherine Noel who, on many occasions, helped me 'clear the fog' and kept my efforts on track to their successful conclusion.

And finally, thanks to my wife and life partner Nancy, without whose love, support and encouragement I could not have completed this monumental project.

Table of Contents

Part Three – Taking Back Control

PREFACE:
SOME PERSONAL PERSPECTIVE

"Adrenaline Nation is a commentary on American culture and how chronic stress is built into the most fundamental aspects of its structure. This stress has led to increases in illness and lower productivity and to our current health care and economic crises. In turn, our response is only creating more stress which then worsens our health and economic systems. We are in a vicious cycle. A perfect storm is forming that will cause it all to come crashing down soon, unless we fix the root cause of this system failure—our culture of stress."

— John Morgenthaler

My personal introduction to the *Adrenaline Nation* and its connection to chronic stress began on May 5, 1961. I was a fifth grade student at Immaculate Heart of Mary grammar school in Scarsdale, NY. That morning, the Sisters of Charity, the teaching order at our school, trooped us all down to the big lunch room in the basement. Mounted high in the corner of the room was a large black-and-white TV, tuned to WCBS-TV in nearby New York City. Sister Lydia, the wall-eyed sixth grade teacher, strode to the front of the room and admonished us, *"Be quiet! You're going to see history made today!"* Just then, the television displayed a close up shot of a black conical shape perched atop a large rocket, which was spewing vapor from its side. That shape was the Mercury spacecraft *Freedom 7*, and strapped inside was Navy Commander Alan Shepard, soon to be the first American to fly in outer space. The voice of Walter Cronkite announced a resumption in the countdown to liftoff. I was totally hooked.

For a somewhat geeky, uncoordinated, overweight schoolboy, this was the dream job I had been searching for. To fly in *outer space!* As the countdown continued, my absorption with the event, and its significance, grew and grew. I wanted to be the guy on top of that rocket! The powerful symbolism of that day was palpable. It was the beginning of an era where we Americans, as a nation and as individuals, truly believed we could do anything, and I was no exception.

Fast forward to the early afternoon of July 20, 1969. I am now a sophomore cadet at the Air Force Academy, propelled there by my still-burning desire to be an astronaut. Having just arrived home on summer leave, I am ensconced in my Dad's lounge chair in our den; my eyes, ears, mind and heart again glued to the television and the voice of Walter Cronkite. For the next five hours, I would not leave that room, following every move of Apollo 11 through undocking of the lunar lander, powered descent and landing on the surface of the moon, and Neil Armstrong's immortal words, "*That's one small step. . .* "

I believe the major reason why I found myself so entranced by these monumental events in American history was that I had completely internalized the belief that I could do anything. And no surprise considering my influences. Raised in the New York City area and the child of media broadcast professionals, I was surrounded by the latest and greatest of American lifestyle enhancements: rapid transportation and communication, state-of-the-art skyscrapers and houses, and the most technologically advanced nutrition and health care delivery systems. The achievement of landing a man on the moon was just the icing on the cake proving that my dream, and any dream, could be a reality!

But although I, like millions of people across the nation, was caught up in the excitement of our achievements, the unwitting price being exacted on me, and all of us, was one I was only to realize many years later: *STRESS*. The mention of the word now brings a variety of reactions from virtually everyone: a knowing nod of the head, rolling of the eyes, and numerous body language and verbal acknowledgments that we truly know what stress is. But do we *really*? And do we *really* understand the effects and costs of the imposition of stress on our bodies and on our society in 21st Century America?

A culture of high achievement and ambition is usually associated with positive results like a greater acquisition of wealth and the accomplishment of a goal, but the dark side of this kind of culture is the feeling that you can never have enough or be good enough. The watchwords of American culture over the last few decades have become "*never give up*," "*you can always be better*," and "*push harder*." We idolize our heroes and then measure ourselves against them. We compete against our co-workers, friends and neighbors in a keeping-up-with-the-Jones' mentality. We continually strive to have more, to be better and to reach for that American dream. We do all of these things habitually and unconsciously without the recognition that, over time, things will inevitably start to crack and fall apart.

Physiologically, we are equipped with the same adrenaline stress response mechanism of our ancient ancestors. However, we Americans are under a stress load to which our bodies can not adequately respond. The constant striving we experience means a constant adrenaline response, but this energy is a finite resource.

Pushing ourselves hard and overdrawing on this resource leads to a depleted body and, frequently, fatal illness. Multiply this effect by thousands, if not millions of times across our society, and the cumulative effects mushroom into the chronic stress we experience across our society – at work, at school, at home, on the road, virtually everywhere.

The problem is that most of us don't know exactly to what degree stress impacts our lives and, of equal importance, how we can change those factors that negatively affect us. A major reason for this problem is our societal belief that someone else is responsible for our health and well-being, so as individuals, we accept that we have no knowledge or power. This is an example of what Deepak Chopra, MD, in his book *Creating Affluence*, accurately calls "*the hypnosis of social conditioning*," or the unquestioning acceptance of a belief or set of beliefs that may or may not be true. However, the startling truth of the negative impact of this type of unconscious behavior over the last several decades is now coming to light. The experience of chronic stress has caused many of us to awaken to the reality that all is NOT right with our health care system and our societal structure, and that the only way we can change things is to educate and empower ourselves, collectively and as individuals.

This concept of self-empowerment is a cornerstone of my practice as a traditional naturopath, a health care practitioner that specializes in wellness, and has proven its validity throughout my years of working with clients. Only through conscientious application of newly learned information can a person change those behaviors which negatively impact his/her health. In turn, this occurs only when the person is sufficiently *motivated* to change, and takes *action* on recommendations for change. Motivation and action: the twin keys to positive change and growth.

My own journey to self-empowerment really began in the mid-1960s with my introduction to the field of complementary and alternative medicine (CAM), as it is now known, and was initially fueled by the typical desire of any young, athletic male: to be bigger, stronger and faster. Perhaps the most enduring legacy I inherited from my father was an appreciation of the athletic benefits of both strength and cardiovascular fitness training. Dad was also the one who initially pointed me toward the vitamin section of our local drug store, my first step into the world of CAM. However, it became quickly obvious to me that these nutritional supplements had inherent value beyond sports conditioning, such as better mental concentration and improved resistance to common illnesses.

Throughout my tenure at the Air Force Academy, I continued to be attracted to this means of assisting my goals of increased fitness and better health, even though at the time they were not readily available to me. After graduation from the Academy in 1972, making a regular paycheck for the first time as an active duty military pilot, I renewed my quest for better health and found the local drug store in Enid, Oklahoma, near where I was stationed. However, as my knowledge base expanded, I saw that there were other, more effective means of achieving my goals, which led me to investigate the then growing number of health food stores, nearby and across the country, and the higher quality nutritional products they carried. I learned early on that just as with any food product, quality matters when you select and consume nutritional supplements. My never ceasing search for better quality led me to both better supplements and an increased knowledge base.

By the mid-1980's, I was well informed and attempted to share my new-found knowledge with my family, but like most people in similar situations at that time, I was branded the family 'health nut.' The amateur nature of my knowledge was obvious and nobody would take me seriously. At the same time, I began to see both of my parents, members of my extended family, and their circle of friends and acquaintances sicken and die from a variety of illnesses. With the level of health knowledge that I possessed, I tended to look at each of the circumstances surrounding their demises as individual occurrences, causally separate from one another. What I didn't know was that living in the New York metropolitan area, one of the highest stress environments in this country, was connected to all of their illnesses.

In those same years, I also acquired academic training in management and organizational behavior and change, and came to see how Corporate America is caught in a vicious cycle of stress. There is a need to control ever-escalating health care costs and at the same time a need to make employees 'more productive,' but the very act of making them more productive increases their stress, thereby directly contributing to the increase in health care costs! My understanding of stress in America had begun.

Then in 1992, though I had not fulfilled my childhood dream of becoming an astronaut, I retired from a successful 20 year military career and transitioned to working as a pilot for a major commercial airline. With my knowledge of the health benefits of CAM as well as that of the stress in Corporate America, I began to notice the effects of chronic stress on both the employees I worked with and the passengers we served. Each flying day, I saw a constant parade of people board our airplanes, many of them in wheelchairs, suffering from a huge variety of illnesses whose root cause was stress. At the same time, the airline crew members themselves were working in an environment which can arguably be described as one of the most hostile to good health on the planet. It is literally full of stressors at every turn. The results are displayed in the fact that pilots suffer from disproportionately high rates of cancer, especially brain cancer, and that female flight attendants are reportedly a segment of the US population with one of the highest rates of autoimmune disease in this country.

Though serious as this situation was, it took until the late 1990's, after the deaths of my mother in 1987 (from congestive heart failure brought on by morbid obesity), my family members and their friends over the years and finally my father in 1996 (from recurrent prostate cancer caused in part by lifelong smoking), to really complete my journey of self-empowerment. I finally clearly saw the limitations of our conventional medical establishment, essentially powerless to help people survive, much less thrive. Like any child dealing with the loss of one's parents, I grieved, but I also became *motivated* and took *action* to personally stay as healthy as possible and to *not* repeat their experience. As well, due to my awareness that living and working in a high stress environment is a prime factor in illness, I committed myself to helping other people where conventional medicine had let them down.

This desire to help others led to beginning my career as a traditional naturopath in 2003. Traditional naturopaths teach clients to employ natural lifestyle approaches which can facilitate the body's own, innate healing and health maintenance mechanisms. We use a combination of in-depth diet and lifestyle counseling, natural substances such as vitamins, herbs and minerals to fill the body's nutritional gaps, and other non-invasive modalities such as energy work, bioresonance therapy and detoxification to help the body return itself to the path of health.

We do not attempt to diagnose or treat disease, but rather recognize that any sub par health condition has its roots in underlying cumulative and destructive processes. These processes may include, but not be limited to, improper diet, lifestyle and relationship issues, environmental factors such as toxic exposure, or a combination of all of these and many more. These mental, emotional and physiological stressors can lead to a breakdown of the body's defenses and subsequently a breakdown in health.

When a client brings a medical diagnosis to the traditional naturopath's office, it becomes just one data point of many, and not the most important one at that. One of my teachers, Elaine Newkirk, ND, puts it best: we keep asking the question "*why?*" about the condition until we get to the root cause of the problem. Once we discover that root cause, we then address it and give the body the tools to help it heal itself.

I have seen the stress management part of my practice explode into its single largest component. Virtually everyone who walks through my office door, from children to the elderly, exhibits the impact of the stress of contemporary life: children with digestive issues, elderly with biochemical imbalances, and working professionals with energy management issues are just some of the many stress-related conditions I have been confronted with.

As my health knowledge has expanded to the professional level and my quest to know more has continued, I now clearly understand the absolutely critical importance and impact of the body's stress response on a whole host of health concerns, and the factors which impact our ability to stay healthy (or not) in today's society. You hold the result of this knowledge and this quest in your hands.

What can you expect to gain from this book? First and most important, you will get a clearer understanding of what stress is and how chronic, unmitigated stress has definite and considerable costs to our economy and our health. We have truly bought into other aspects of the "hypnosis of social conditioning," that we can easily deal with stress and that the solutions we have chosen, or that have been chosen for us, cheaply and effectively cope with it. Nothing could be further from the truth. The impact of chronic stress goes far beyond the purely personal or familial. The cumulative impact of our institutional, individual and societal reaction to stress is like a pebble dropped in a pond. It ripples throughout virtually every facet of our civilization: our work, our health, our relationships, our spirituality, and our economy.

The second learning objective I offer in this book is a better understanding of our bodies' reaction to stress, and the pervasive influence this reaction has on virtually every aspect of our lives. This is important from an individual standpoint, as well as from an organizational management standpoint. Responsible corporate managers need to become more fully aware that the demands placed on their employees generate definite and considerable costs to their corporations' bottom lines. Although we as a society continue to pride ourselves on our increasing technological and cultural sophistication, our physiology has not changed appreciably in millennia. The environment in which we live today could not be more different than the prehistoric era in which we evolved. It is this widening gap between the finite capabilities of our physiological reactions and the demands of the environment to which we react that is at the root of most of our contemporary health problems and, therefore, of the dilemma in which American society finds itself.

Third and finally, this book provides a step-by-step plan for individuals and organizations to take back control and move into action to benefit both themselves and those around them. This knowledge is essential to empower our choices and affect a powerful change in our businesses, our individual lives, our families, and our overarching societal structures. It is the cornerstone of an important campaign to bring this awareness to both the business community and the general public. Once we have the facts, we can all take responsibility to alter our course in order to protect and improve our finances, quality of life, state of health and overall well being. *Adrenaline Nation* is an urgent and compelling wake up call for our stressed-out economy, population and society.

At this point, you should offer yourself a pat on the back. By being motivated to pick up this book and begin to read it, you are taking a powerful, life changing step towards improving your -- and our entire society's -- reaction to and ability to handle the stressors which are imposed upon us. I would ask you to do me one favor: if, after you have finished this book, you feel that it has value, take action. Not only implement the recommendations yourself, but help our society better deal with stress and tell at least two friends about it. Only by increasing the awareness of our fellow citizens will we be able to make a lasting difference in how we deal with stress, both individually and as a society.

Live Peacefully,

Peter McCarthy
Traditional Naturopath

Part One

Living and Working with The Stress Stack:

Benefits and Costs

CHAPTER 1

WHAT IS STRESS?

"Every human being is the author of his own health or disease."

— *Swami Sivananda, 1887-1963*

Chronic stress is, slowly but surely, compromising our citizens' health, bankrupting our government, and ruining Corporate America's bottom line. And despite well educated and intentioned government officials and health care professionals, an incredibly productive workforce, and a fiscally mindful business community, America has not been able to solve this vexing, multidimensional problem. So it is clear that we must first look at the root cause of it by answering the question: what exactly is stress?

At the outset, it is important to note that not all stress is harmful. Hans Selye, MD, considered the father of stress research, called the so-called 'good' stress *"eustress,"* a type of stress that enhances physical or mental function. Examples of this type of stress are strength training, any type of aerobic exercise, or work that one finds stimulating or challenging. In contrast, Selye described *"distress"* as the type of stress that does not resolve itself through an adaptive response, i.e., an appropriate reaction to an environmental demand, and results in negative physical, mental or emotional consequences. It is this type of stress that most people think of when they define the term *"chronic stress."*

Ask a group of people of any size the question above; while you may get common agreement on some stressors, when you boil it down to the individual particulars, everyone has a somewhat different definition of stress. This makes perfect sense, given the individual and unique nature of each of our bodies. Since 1956, when the respected biochemist Roger J. Williams demonstrated that we are each biochemically unique, the scientific community has acknowledged that as fact. It stands to reason, therefore, that our view of stress, and therefore our response to it, would be unique also.

Actually, the differentiation is made with respect to both *the identified stressors* and *the results of their imposition*. While one person cites work-related stress, another may cite family pressures, still another may indicate classroom-related stress, and the list goes on. At the same time, some people may indicate that the primary effect of stress is mental, some physical, and others emotional, or some combination of all three. In order to provide you with a complete yet understandable definition of the concept of stress, I embarked on a brief journey of exploration and education which I will share with you here.

To begin with, Webster's dictionary defines stress as "*A state resulting from a stress; especially one of bodily or mental tension resulting from factors that tend to alter an existent equilibrium.*" Sounds pretty good, but the language is somewhat imprecise and incomplete in its description of a phenomenon that is so widely and variably experienced.

Approaching it from a more clinically oriented point of view, *Mosby's Medical Encyclopedia* offered some additional insights. Mosby's defined stress as "*any emotional, physical, social, economic, or other factor that requires a response or change, as severe loss of fluid, which can cause a rise in body temperature, or a separation from parents, which can cause a young child to cry.*" It further defined stress behavior as "*a change from a person's normal behavior in response to something that causes wear and tear on the body's physical or mental resources (stressor).*"

Mosby's cross referenced to a condition called *general adaptation syndrome (GAS), or adaptation syndrome.* This was first identified by Hans Selye in 1936 and defined as "*the defense response of the body or mind to injury or prolonged stress. It begins with a stage of shock or alarm, followed by resistance or adaptation, and ending in either a state of adjustment and healing or of exhaustion and disintegration.*"

We're getting closer, but there is still a frustrating lack of specificity. Not satisfied with either Webster's or Mosby's definitions, I went to the Worldwide Web to see if there were other perspectives on stress. Were there ever!

The Free Dictionary web site offered definitions applicable to both physics and medicine. The physics definition specified stress as an "*applied force or system of forces that tends to strain or deform a body*" and "*internal resistance of a body to such an applied force or system of forces.*" Once again, a somewhat concise but non-specific definition, having in common with both Webster and Mosby's the concepts that stress is both a stimulus and the result of that stimulus.

The medically oriented definition went one step further, calling stress "*a mentally or emotionally disruptive or upsetting condition occurring in response to adverse external influences and capable of affecting physical health, usually characterized by increased heart rate, a rise in blood pressure, muscular tension, irritability, and depression,*" plus "*a stimulus or circumstance causing such a condition.*" An additional dimension was offered: "*A state of extreme difficulty, pressure, or strain.*" So we now must incorporate the additional dimension of specific physiological manifestations associated with stress, plus a decidedly negative undertone (i.e., that stress is somehow bad or harmful).

I also checked Wikipedia since it is one of the most popular websites for free information. Their definition of stress is "*a medical term for a wide range of strong external stimuli, both physiological and psychological, which can cause the physiological response called the 'general adaptation syndrome,' first described in 1936 by Hans Selye in the journal Nature.*" Wikipedia has the added benefit of offering a section of its site for user comments. This definition and its accompanying article, a relatively small portion of the overall Wikipedia data base, nevertheless elicited quite a few interesting and insightful comments from both lay people and health professionals alike.

For example, one commentator remarked that "*'roughly the opposite of relaxation' is a pretty good approximation [of the definition of stress], I suppose.*" Another commented that "*the article never distinguishes between positive stress and negative stress, just that the two different types exist. In fact, I was under the impression that all stress is bad.*" Again, we see a negative connotation attached to stress. In contrast, someone else observed "*that what appear to others to be purely positive events can cause stress to particular individuals because of the way they react or perceive the events -- this can be because of personal history, phobias and/or the inability to deal with new situations in an appropriate fashion.*"

Here was a new perspective! Other factors besides the purely physiological can impact a person's response to stress. The variability of the stress response was highlighted by another commentator who summarized, "*Stress is something we all understand intuitively but is hard to define. While many studies link 'stress' (note the quotation marks!) to various illnesses such as cardiovascular disease, absence from work, and total mortality, the definition of stress in each study is different, and based on a different set of tests. We should report results of studies based on their detailed definitions, even though those vary.*" I detected again some intermingling here between the actual stressors and the results of the imposition of those stressors, but his central point is valid. The type, amount, duration, intensity and degree of normalization of the stress response are ALL variables in any study addressing stress.

Apparently, some segments of the health care community took exception to Wikipedia's definition. Paul J. Rosch, MD, FACP, Clinical Professor of Medicine and Psychiatry at New York Medical College, President of The American Institute of Stress, and Honorary Vice President of the International Stress Management Association affirmed that "*stress is not the opposite of relaxation. It is, as originally defined by Hans Selye, 'the non-specific response of the body to any demand for change.'*"

Wikipedia rightly recognizes that Dr. Rosch served a fellowship with Hans Selye (considered the trailblazer in stress research) in 1951 and was a close professional colleague and friend of Selye throughout his life. Rosch also served as Editor in Chief of *Stress Medicine* and has been involved in stress research for well over a half century with numerous publications on various stress related subjects. However, "*the non-specific response of the body to any demand for change*" is, from a layperson's perspective, still very hazy in its description.

Other health care professionals have also attempted to weigh in on this subject. From the web site MedicineNet.com, Medical Editor Leslie J. Schoenfield, MD, PhD and his colleague Peter J. Pazarino, MD, FAPA, offer that "*stress is simply a fact of nature -- forces from the outside world affecting the individual.*" In their article, they go on to assert that "*from a biological point of view, stress can be neutral, negative, or positive.*" They also tie their definition into the evolution of life on Earth, affirming that "*the species that adapted best to the causes of stress (stressors) have survived and evolved into the plant and animal kingdoms we now observe.*" So now we have an aspect of stress that includes our bodies' survival mechanisms.

A final interesting perspective came from TimeThoughts.com, a web site catering to business professionals, offering "*resources for personal and career success.*" Their contribution? "*Researchers define stress as a physical, mental, or emotional response to events that causes bodily or mental tension. Simply put, stress is any outside force or event that has an effect on our body or mind.*" This is but one example of the many that I found which document the business world's significant interest in and concern about stress.

But What IS Stress? As you can clearly see, there are as many definitions of stress as there are people, regardless of their professional expertise. Some emphasize the stressors themselves, some the results. Some try to incorporate their own experience into the definition, some to use the most sophisticated scientific tools that are available.

There are two interesting commonalities with all of these: first, they are *all* correct from their personal or professional perspective; second, they all address only a small portion of the definition of stress. It is literally as if each observer/commentator is looking at a small corner of a very large painting, and attempting to describe the subject of that painting from the information obtained from that very small corner.

It became obvious to me that to derive an accurate and comprehensive definition of stress, one that is usable for everyone, I had to incorporate all these apparently competing ideas into an understandable whole. In order to do so, I also had to identify the common denominator in all these definitions, the thing to which each refers, either directly or indirectly. When I compared all of these varying concepts of stress, those which stimulate stress and those which emanate from stress, the common denominator came clearly into focus for me. What's the common denominator? The stress response, also commonly known as the fight-or-flight response, functions to help us survive in the face of threats.

To be more specific, the fight-or-flight response is a primordial, autonomic (automatic) survival mechanism whose functioning is the body's way of marshaling its energy resources to either escape or confront threats to its survival, and has been unchanged in humans for many thousands of years. Were we to travel back in time, standing beside our ancient ancestor facing down a saber tooth cat on a forest trail, our bodies' responses would be essentially the same. The difference between us and the humans of that time is that today there is a yawning gap between this ability of the human body to respond to stress and the stress load placed upon it. Said another way, we 21st century humans are equipped with a prehistoric stress response, as well as the limitations that entails, but are exposed to an almost constant imposition of various stressors from a myriad of directions.

What limitations? Though every living being on this planet continues to exist because it is able to produce energy to sustain that existence, we are all finite beings, therefore our available sources of energy for the tasks of living are, by definition, also finite. There is only so much available at any given time.

Look at it this way: when you go to the market to buy your groceries, you usually write a check, pay cash, or use a debit or credit card, right? The common element is that any of these four means of payment involve *finite* resources. The check or debit card draw from the available balance in your checking account; the cash from the money in your wallet; the credit card from the finite credit limit made available by the bank that issued it.

The human body operates in much the same way: any activity in which it engages, or internal process by which it operates, is constrained by the availability of its *finite* energy resources. Similarly, just as an overdraw of one's checking account or exceeding one's credit card limit can have an adverse impact on one's financial health, overdrawing your body's finite energy resources, especially through chronic stress, *will* adversely impact your physical health.

So how does that impact the definition of "*stress?*" By incorporating all of the previous concepts, we can accurately state that *stress is any input to the human physiology that expends the body's finite energy resources on activation of the fight-or-flight response, as well as the resulting effects of those inputs.*

The Stress Stack: A New Concept in Managing Stress. While most people clearly understand the explanations above, what has been missing from the discussion until now has been a way for people to understand how all the stressors we have discussed fit together and react with the human body, and how those factors have an impact on our health. The goal is to integrate the concepts we have just discussed with the experiences of our daily lives.

Because every human being is biologically unique, the mix of stressors that impact their lives is also unique. Therefore, any explanation or depiction of this process must allow for the expression of that uniqueness. To accomplish this, I have derived a model called 'The Stress Stack' to help us better understand these complex interrelationships.

Understanding The Stress Stack. The key to understanding 'The Stress Stack' is to first understand its characteristics. As individuals, we each accumulate our own unique set of life stressors which are in a constant state of flux, stacking up like building blocks, or stacks of firewood, and increasing in size until they become unmanageable. As a result, each individual's Stress Stack displays unique, dynamic, cumulative and holistic characteristics.

For example, if you are a corporate office worker, you likely are continuously exposed to a high level of electronic equipment radiation, perhaps a daily dose or doses of caffeinated beverages, one or more servings of high calorie, fat-laden foods, and maybe a pattern of chronic sleep deprivation. On the other hand, if you are an agricultural worker, you may be exposed to high levels of chemical fertilizers and, if you smoke, to the effects of cigarette smoke. Each of these examples, and more too numerous to count, create an *individual* set of stressors in each category, and therefore an individual Stress Stack.

When you review the individual blocks of the Stress Stack, you will see that the inputs to each of the blocks varies continually over time. This in turn results in continual changes in both the size of each block and their effects on your body. Again using the example of the corporate office worker, the effect of each of the factors mentioned above will vary based on the frequency and duration of exposure. The same can be said of the agricultural worker, or anyone else for that matter. The Stress Stack is constantly in motion, with the inputs to and effect of each block continually varying over time.

However, the effects of each block are always cumulative, unless you take positive action to reduce their effects. In *Caffeine Blues*, Stephen Cherniski discusses the 'vacation illusion,' the perception that 'a couple of weeks off' will completely alleviate your stress and leave you good as new.

In reality, unless you take major positive action to deal decisively with the causes of stress as contained in your personal Stress Stack, the 'vacation reality' will result in simply a delay of the inevitable crossing into the zone where progressively more destructive changes in your body will ultimately result in the descent into overt illness.

Perhaps most important is your understanding that chronic stress is a holistic phenomenon. In this fast food-oriented society with its emphasis on easy, quick fixes, we tend to gravitate to anything that seems rapid and simple. However, recovering from the effects of chronic stress is neither. The conditions that have created your Stress Stack have, in most cases, taken years to develop to their current state. Equally important, those conditions were very likely created by the influence of several factors working together simultaneously, so reliance on one or two actions, remedies or therapies to address the problem will likely not do the job. Rather, they will typically lull one into a misguided sense of complacency and merely delay the inevitable day of reckoning.

The First Block: Foods and Beverages That Cause Stress. When ingested by the human body, these are the substances which cause either a direct or indirect activation of the body's stress response. They include caffeine, artificial sweeteners, processed sugar, white flour, and trans fats. The first block of the Stress Stack therefore looks like this:

Dietary Influences (Foods and Beverages Which Cause Stress)	Caffeine, Artificial Sweeteners, Processed Sugar, White Flour, Trans Fats

Why are these particular items included in this first block? Let's start with caffeine. We have been positively inundated with messages in the popular media about the supposed benefits of caffeine, the world's most popular stimulant: more energy; better, more intense workouts; better elimination; quicker weight loss; the antioxidant content of coffee, the list goes on. A closer look reveals a far different picture.

When it arrives in the stomach, caffeine starts a reaction as if the stomach had just received a large portion of protein, causing the secretion of both hydrochloric acid and protein digesting enzymes. If there is nothing for this acid-enzyme combination to react with, the combination can eventually damage the stomach itself. That is why so many chronic caffeine users (abusers, really) develop stomach problems such as ulcers.

As it continues into the digestive tract, caffeine kills much of the intestinal flora (or 'good' bacteria, e.g., acidophilus, lactobacillus, etc.) needed by the body for proper food processing. This sets the stage for long-term digestive problems. Without the proper balance of intestinal flora in the digestive tract, any food passing through will not be properly broken down and can putrefy, causing a major increase in the body's toxic and stress loads.

Entering the bloodstream, caffeine depletes significant amounts of Vitamins B and C, and many important minerals such as potassium. The B vitamins allow the central nervous system to deal effectively with various forms of stress, the very thing most caffeine users cite when they justify their own caffeine use ("*I need caffeine to cope!*"). The C vitamins are contained in high concentrations in the adrenal glands themselves, and are used to support a host of adrenal-related functions that are critical to an effective stress response. Ironically, the consumption of caffeine actually makes the body less able to deal with stress. It causes the body to remain in the 'fight-or-flight' response mode, as if it were continually facing a physical threat to its survival.

As part of this response, caffeine over stimulates the adrenal glands, causing the rapid heart rate associated with the 'caffeine rush.' Over time, chronic usage can actually exhaust the adrenal glands, causing fatigue, hampered immune response, and heartbeat irregularities. The secretion of adrenaline (also known as epinephrine) and its subsequent absence is why many chronic caffeine users feel more tired after caffeine consumption than before ingestion (the infamous 'caffeine crash'), thus needing more and more caffeine to remain 'energized.' It's literally like beating a dead horse.

At the same time, caffeine dramatically increases the body's secretion of cortisol, a hormone the body uses to deal with stress, in particular, pain and inflammation. Chronic caffeine overuse has also recently been implicated in the onset of several serious chronic diseases, such as fibrocystic breast disease, several different types of cancer, autoimmune disorders, heart disease and osteoporosis.

Caffeine also accelerates destruction of glucosamine in the body's cartilage. When our bodies are younger, this does not have an immediate impact because the body is still able to manufacture its own glucosamine. Starting at around age 40, however, the body gradually stops manufacturing its own replacement glucosamine. Any cartilage destroyed by caffeine at this time is permanently lost unless replaced by nutritional supplementation. It therefore makes perfect sense that we don't take our glucosamine supplements with our morning coffee!

And then there's chocolate. I know there are many people reading this right now that are reacting with "*oh, no, not my chocolate!*" Believe me, I've seen the T-shirts in mail order catalogs with the caption "*Hand Over The Chocolate And No One Gets Hurt!*" I know what this food holds in terms of emotional contentment; it is a preeminent 'comfort food.' Unfortunately, it is sad but true: yes, chocolate! Two substances in chocolate, caffeine and theobromine, combine to make a three ounce chocolate candy bar the equivalent, caffeine-wise, of a large mug of coffee.

Long-term studies also show that continued caffeine usage decreases bone mineral density in women, who are at higher risk for osteoporosis as they age. (These studies only looked at women, but the results are equally applicable to men!). Additionally, caffeine is a powerful diuretic, causing the body to excrete more water by volume than the amount of caffeine consumed. Since most people do not consume enough water as it is, this adds dramatically to the problem of dehydration, currently experienced by over 60 per cent of the American population.

Finally, when caffeine crosses the blood-brain barrier, it attacks the choline in the brain. Choline is intimately tied to the brain's memory retention processes. Long-term use of caffeine has been shown to detrimentally impact memory.

Many habitual caffeine users cite the feeling of alertness and focus caffeine gives them as justification for continued use. In reality, extensive research has revealed that the 'fight-or-flight' reflex stimulated by caffeine significantly degrades the functioning of the creative, judgmental and decision making portions of the brain. Recent research has also shown that when caffeine enters the brain it causes the release of the adrenal hormone cortisol which helps decrease insulin sensitivity in the body. When insulin sensitivity decreases, blood sugar is less available to the cells of the body for producing energy. This is particularly detrimental to people with diabetes.

Given all of the above, can there be any doubt that caffeine is a source of stress?

Next, let's examine the artificial sweetener aspartame, currently the one in widest use. Does aspartame really live up to its billing as an aid to weight loss? Despite its approval by the Food and Drug Administration (FDA), is aspartame a truly safe product? A look at its effects paints a very sobering picture.

To start with, aspartame is approximately 180 times as sweet as sugar, but with zero calorie content. Although billed as an advantage over sugar, these chemical properties alone cause many of the problems aspartame creates. When the body ingests and identifies a substance this sweet, it instructs the intestinal tract to prepare for an enormous intake of calories. The body creates enzymes to convert future calories to fat. This process is called 'cephalic phase response.' It programs the liver to stop converting protein and carbohydrates to energy and instead instructs it to transform the nutrients into fat for storage. Because aspartame is so intensely sweet, and because its effect on appetite lasts for up to 90 minutes after ingestion, it causes an overwhelming urge to overeat. That is why the more aspartame one ingests, the more likely they are to gain weight. Look at it this way: how many thin people do you know who drink diet soda? In actual fact, not many.

Once the aspartame is actually in the bloodstream, even more damage occurs. Above 86 degrees F. (about 12 degrees below the normal body temperature of 98.6 degrees), aspartame breaks down into its chemical components of phenylalanine, aspartate and methanol.

Phenylalanine is an amino acid which competes for absorption in the brain with the amino acid tryptophan. Tryptophan is crucial for maintaining the serotonin levels necessary for stable mood. The phenylalanine in aspartame blocks the action of tryptophan, thus creating an insufficiency in the brain which has been closely linked to illnesses such as depression. Recent research has also tied tryptophan insufficiency to the development of diabetes and cell mutation. In fact, largely because of this information, Dr. H.J. Roberts, the world's leading expert on aspartame, identified it as a diabetic reactor and neurotoxin and advises all his diabetes patients to avoid aspartame products.

Phenylalanine also lowers the seizure threshold in the brain and, in combination with lower serotonin levels, may predispose a person to erratic, unusual or even violent behavior. Of equal significance, according to Dr. Louis Elsas, Pediatrician/Professor of Genetics, Emory University, in his testimony before Congress, phenylalanine can concentrate in the placenta of a developing fetus, causing fetal mental retardation.

Aspartate also significantly damages the body. Like phenylalanine, aspartate is a highly excitatory neurotransmitter. When consumed in large quantities (like those found in diet drinks), these two chemicals act together to change the basic activity level of the brain to an unhealthy, constantly stimulated state. When caffeine is added to the mix, the effect is greatly increased. Even more serious, as Dr. Batmanghelidj (see the Resources section for his important book) states, "*receptors for aspartate are abundantly present on some nerve systems whose products also stimulate the reproductive organs and breasts. A constant stimulation of breast glands without the other factors associated with pregnancy may well be implicated in the rise in the rate of breast cancer in women.*" Finally, aspartate causes indiscriminate overuse of the energy cells of the brain, causing thirst/hunger to replace the lost energy reserves, and literally killing the brain cells in the process.

However, perhaps the most dangerous component of aspartame is methanol, also known as wood alcohol, and already well known as a killer and blinder of countless homeless people on skid row. The EPA recommends consumption of no more than 7.8mg/day of methanol, but an average aspartame-sweetened soft drink produces 56mg. Once ingested, the methanol converts to formaldehyde and formic acid (ant sting poison). Formaldehyde, a deadly neurotoxin, is common embalming fluid, a Class A carcinogen.

Up until 2007, one of the less explored complications of aspartame was its effect as a possible facilitator in cancer formation. However, that question has been put convincingly to rest by two studies conducted by researchers at the European Ramazzini Institute in Italy. In an April 2007 presentation before doctors and researchers at Mt. Sinai Hospital in New York City, primary researcher Dr. Morando Soffritti rebutted critics of the Institute's initial study to show that aspartame does, indeed, cause cancer in laboratory animals. For his team's groundbreaking research, Dr. Soffritti received Mt. Sinai's prestigious Irving J. Selikoff Award.

The symptoms that many habitual aspartame consumers eventually develop can mimic multiple sclerosis, when in reality the problem is methanol toxicity. When the victim discontinues consumption of aspartame, most of the symptoms disappear. In cases of systemic lupus, which is triggered by aspartame, the victim usually does not know that the aspartame is the culprit. In some cases, the victim continues its use, aggravating the lupus to such a degree that it can become life threatening. Those people with systemic lupus who cease using the product usually become asymptomatic. Unfortunately, the disease cannot be reversed. In the case of diabetics, the methanol can accumulate in the retina of the eye, causing symptoms of diabetic retinopathy; again, in reality the cause is methanol toxicity.

Of significance to women wishing to become pregnant, Dr. Roberts adds that,"*consuming aspartame at the time of conception can cause birth defects*." Fetal tissue cannot tolerate methanol and Dr. James Bowen calls aspartame instant birth control. When you think about it a minute that makes perfect sense: how can you expect to create new life in an environment containing a chemical which is designed to preserve *dead* tissue?

In summary, aspartame is *definitely* a source of stress when ingested.

Next, let's examine the effects of white flour and processed sugar. Many people are well familiar with the 'sugar high' that they experience when they eat high sugar foods. The same can be said about the effects of foods made with white flour. The common element in both is that, once they are digested and enter the bloodstream, they exert almost identical effects on the body.

How does that relate to stress? Very simply, each type of food is converted into large amounts of glucose. The body's ability to process that glucose depends in large part upon the ability of the adrenal glands to secrete adequate amounts of cortisol, also known as glucocorticoid. The larger the amount of glucose in the bloodstream, the greater the demand on the adrenals, and the more profound the level of stress.

At the same time, the pancreas secretes another hormone called insulin to allow the body to use the glucose effectively. Again, the greater the amount of glucose in the bloodstream, the greater the amount of insulin is required to process it.

The practical effect of such large amounts of glucose in the bloodstream is threefold. First, it creates the conditions that lead to the previously mentioned 'sugar high.' But since such large amounts of cortisol and insulin are introduced into the bloodstream so rapidly, they help to so rapidly process the glucose that the blood sugar levels fluctuate wildly, zooming up rapidly at first, but then plummeting just as rapidly and resulting in the now infamous 'sugar crash.'

The third effect, though more subtle, is even more detrimental. When a person habitually engages in this behavior, perhaps several times a day, for weeks, months or years on end, it can literally wear out both the adrenal glands and the pancreas. This can set the stage for serious illnesses such as Addison's disease (the complete cessation of adrenal function), diabetes, or other serious disorders. We will discuss these unpleasant results in detail in a later chapter.

The last dietary influence is trans fats. By now, most Americans are aware that trans fats are detrimental to their health, and that high concentrations of trans fats are a major contributing factor to heart disease, as well high cholesterol and high triglyceride levels in the bloodstream. That awareness has precipitated the introduction of a wide array of food products that are labeled 'zero trans fats,' or something similar. But there is an equally important, less well known detriment to high trans fat consumption, one that directly impacts the body's ability to respond to stress.

When we examine the basic biochemical processes that the body undergoes while responding to stress, we discover that one of the key chemical reactions occurs when essential fatty acids (EFAs), otherwise known as Omega-3s, bind to specific receptor sites on the cell membrane. These EFAs serve a number of functions in the body, not least of which is serving as the raw material from which the adrenal hormones, cortisol and DHEA, are formed. They also play key roles in maintaining brain health and cardiovascular health.

Unfortunately, though, ingestion of trans fats short circuits the cell receptor binding process mentioned above. Because of their unique chemical composition, trans fats are more strongly attracted to these cell receptor sites than are EFAs. Said another way, if the cell receptor has a choice between latching onto an EFA molecule or a trans fat molecule, the trans fat molecule will win every time. The result is that the trans fats sabotage the cellular functions meant to be completed by the EFAs, leading to an impaired stress response. It's a lot like asking your gasoline powered car to run on diesel fuel; you can put diesel in your gas tank, but your car won't run for long with that kind of fuel. In this respect, we must count trans fats among the dietary influences on the body's stress response.

The Second Block: Lifestyle Influences. There are a whole host of factors in our society, and therefore our daily lives, which impact our bodies' ability to respond to and withstand stress. Many of these factors have become so ingrained in our society that they are widely accepted as 'normal.' As mentioned previously, Deepak Chopra, MD calls this phenomenon "*the hypnosis of social conditioning.*"

In Corporate America, the level of stress has risen dramatically over the last several decades. With its dual emphasis on quality and quantity, Corporate America has placed a stress load on corporate employees which is unprecedented in human history.

At the same time, the natural friction between the desires of corporations to provide good service and maintain operational cost effectiveness has foisted a much greater workload on the customer, in terms of time spent interacting with the corporation over issues such as product problems and service. When the perception is created that the corporation's money is more important than the customer's time, customer stress is generated.

In major metropolitan areas, the daily stress of traffic congestion adds immeasurably to the commuter's stress load. Using road systems designed for the 'average' traffic flow, commuters suffer through the daily mess caused by accidents and the overwhelming of the infrastructure by too many vehicles in too little space. When you consider the fact that the average American drives to and from work 5 days a week, 50 weeks a year, over a 40 year working lifetime, you realize their exposure to this stressor alone creates the potential of about 20,000 stressful events, some which may be hours in length.

In most cities, corporate office buildings are typically multistory or high rise, steel framed buildings with central climate control. Therein lie two of Corporate America's most widely experienced but least recognized stressors.

To understand why this is so, we need to first recognize that, at our most fundamental level, we are all energetic beings. Each of us produces and radiates a low level electromagnetic field that interfaces with and reacts to the electromagnetic environment around us. One characteristic of this field is that it causes our DNA to vibrate at the speed of about 7.8 cycles per second, or Hertz (Hz). This also happens to be the same average rate at which Earth's electromagnetic field vibrates.

Under normal circumstances, little of what we experience, or are exposed to, will alter that vibration substantially or permanently. However, when we walk into a steel framed office building, we enter the equivalent of a metal cage environment that has a profound effect on our field.

Richard Gerber, MD, in his ground breaking book *Vibrational Medicine for the 21st Century*, cites this influence as a possible explanation for the prevalence of the mysterious 'sick building syndrome' that has afflicted countless corporate employees around the country.

Certainly, one-time or infrequent exposure to this environment is obviously not harmful. But an examination of the American corporate worker's typical working lifetime permits us to gage the true effect of this exposure. If we recognize again that most people in this environment work at least 8 hours a day, 5 days a week, 50 weeks a year, over 40 years, they are exposed to at least 80,000 hours of this environment. It is the consistent exposure to this environment, and the resulting consistent distortion of the body's vibrational field at the DNA level, that causes problems. It cannot help but distort critical cell functions and processes, and therefore the operation of the body's systems which are comprised of those cells.

The prevalence of stressful content on TV and in the mainstream media (e.g., violent programming, negative news stories) also creates a stress response. In many cases, the content is so stimulating that an accompanying emotional response (e.g., fear, shock, etc.) is also generated. The widespread use of technology in American homes and workplaces also generates its own kind of stress. Long-term exposure to the electrical fields generated by home and workplace appliances and computers is increasingly being recognized as harmful.

As our society has become progressively more automated, our personal relationships, at home and at work, have become more fragmented. The gradually increasing isolation of most Americans, despite their ever increasing electronic connectedness, has created an epidemic of loneliness. Research has recently identified loneliness as a primary factor in the body's inability to mount an effective stress response.

As mentioned earlier, despite our apparently sophisticated civilization, our body's stress response operates in essentially the same way as our ancestors. As such, we still need regular exercise to help our bodies normalize their stress responses. However, the advent of myriad labor saving devices, which impact virtually every area of our lives, has created another "*hypnosis of social conditioning*" which has convinced too many of our fellow citizens that exercise is merely an option in pursuing good health. As such, they deny themselves one of the most important and readily available remedies to combat a chronic stress response.

One of the most widespread stressors in American life is sleep deprivation. With the virtually endless options available for nighttime entertainment, as well as the desire of Corporate America to increase worker productivity, we have truly become a 24/7 Society. The physiological costs to those of us who routinely deny themselves adequate rest add significantly to our stress load.

When we incorporate these factors into the Stress Stack, we now have a stack of two blocks that look like this:

Dietary Influences (Foods and Beverages Which Cause Stress)	Caffeine, Artificial Sweeteners, Processed Sugar, White Flour, Trans Fats
Lifestyle Influences (Activities and Habits Which Cause Stress)	Driving in Traffic, Inactivity, Sleep Deprivation, Relationships

The Third Block: Our Own 'Cognitive Filter'. Of all the stressors which impact the human body/mind/spirit matrix, though, perhaps the most influential is what I call the 'cognitive filter.' It is the overlay of influences and experiences through which we perceive, interpret and act upon the events which shape our reality. By events, I mean the combination of mental activity (i.e., thoughts) and physical action which we generate, take or experience throughout our lives.

There is some Nobel Prize-winning research which supports this contention. In 1977, Drs. Guillemin and Schalley proved that thoughts and mind pictures can be translated into hormone secretions in the body. The old adage of "*you are what you eat*" has a new partner: "*you are what you think.*"

In order to best understand how our cognitive filters work, we need to know how our bodies work to generate those filters. Perhaps the closest equivalent which has already been described is the 'life grid' concept developed by British physician Leon Chaitow. Although originally derived as a tool for physicians to describe the symptom patterns, causes and effects of the disease fibromyalgia, with some modification it can be used more generally. This is because a major part of the symptomology of fibromyalgia, as well as many other autoimmune disorders, involves the inability to manage the stress response, either physiologically or psychologically.

While most stressed people don't suffer from these diseases, the processes at work are the same; they just haven't progressed to the point where an overt disease state exists. I would be remiss if I did not offer a word of thanks to Dr. Chaitow for developing the 'life grid.' Because of his work, we have now been able to derive a comprehensive model with which to explain our behavior under stress.

Chaitow describes his model as "*a series of 'grids' through which the individual can be viewed, each of which adds a number of variables to the complex combination which each person represents, made up of their unique genetic, biochemical, biomechanical and psychological features . . .*"

To his list I would add the spiritual component, since it typically plays at least as large a role in determining one's perception of reality, and by implication the nature of one's stress response, as any of the other factors mentioned.

What exactly is a 'life grid?' The baseline factors are comprised first of the individual's current and past biochemical stressors. These can include not only the various toxic influences which impact one's long-term health (e.g., mercury in the dental fillings or fluoride in the drinking water), but also those near term influences such as the food we eat, the cosmetics we use, the beverages we drink, etc. It has been stated on more than one occasion, and by more than one scholar, that every substance we ingest, absorb, breathe, etc. has a pharmacological effect on our bodies, minds and spirits. These subjects alone would comprise several additional books. One must also include the effect of current and past exposure to drugs, be they prescription, over-the-counter or recreational (yes, alcohol and caffeine are included!).

Besides the actual biochemical effects of these substances, one must also account for their energetic influences. Since we have been conclusively proven to be energetic beings, with a measurable electromagnetic field, we must also accept the fact that any substance we ingest or absorb also has an energetic effect on our bodies.

The homeopathy concept of the 'miasm' plays a very important role here. A 'miasm' is an energetic signature of a given influence, imprinted at the cellular and/or genetic level. The genesis of these imprints can be either physiological or psychological in nature, or a combination of both.

When dealing with toxic influences especially, one must be prepared to deal with the toxicity at both the biochemical and energetic levels. To do less would permit the individual to achieve biochemical balance, only to suffer a relapse because the miasmic imprint of the ailment allows it to be first energetically and then biochemically reestablished. This is a possible and plausible explanation for the high incidence of recurrence of cancers of various kinds. While Western medicine sometimes does a credible job of altering the biochemical balance, the energetic balance is virtually ignored.

The second input variable is the current and past psychological load. This would be comprised of the totality from birth of one's thoughts and mental and emotional reactions as stored in the brain. Obviously, repetitive patterns (be they positive or negative), as imprinted within the brain structure, would have a much greater influence than discrete events, unless those individual events were overlaid with exceptionally strong emotional content. Once again, any 'hypnoses of social conditioning' that we have either been taught or learned through experience will exert exceptionally powerful influence, especially in the emotional arena. I'll address the powerful effects of emotion on health in a later chapter.

The third input is current and past biomechanical overuse and misuse. All of us suffer from this inadequacy to some degree. Since none of us are structurally perfect, we must compensate for our flaws by overuse of some components and under use of others. When injury and illness are overlaid, the tendencies are exacerbated, creating visible imbalances and manifestations.

One of my teachers, Dr. Heith Root, DC, is a veritable master of assessing the location and severity of these imbalances and, equally important, taking action to correct them. Another teacher, Adrian Keller, a master Rolfer, can spot musculoskeletal imbalances from simply observing one's posture. Their expertise points up the fact that such imbalances can and should be addressed. However, the equally important point is that these influences can create very strong and influential self-perceptions and self-limitations, thus significantly influencing the cognitive filter.

The fourth input is the spiritual component. Many of us have chosen not to acknowledge this aspect of ourselves, either because we have mistakenly equated spirituality with religion (and choose not to participate), or because our understanding of our world does not acknowledge this dimension of existence. I believe this is a very narrow viewpoint that we espouse at great potential detriment to ourselves.

By that I do *not* mean detriment in the 'hellfire and brimstone,' religiously oriented sense of the word, but in the sense of divorcing ourselves from being part of something much larger and more significant than us as individuals, and therefore depriving ourselves of the opportunity to make a much larger contribution to our world than we presently believe we are capable of making.

One of my friends and teachers in this area, Gwen Jones, simply but powerfully describes this concept as the 'big work' we have all been created to accomplish. Unfortunately, many of us never achieve the level of awareness necessary to complete this 'big work.'

However, it should be emphasized that each one of us possesses a different level and comprehension of the concept of 'spiritual awareness.' *None* of these differences is right, wrong, good or bad. They are all different and unique. A given level of awareness may be completely fulfilling and satisfying to one person, but cause another to embark on a decades-long quest for increased understanding.

The primary point here is that we must all recognize that we *each* have a unique, individualized level of spiritual awareness, and it can play either a positive or negative role in our lives with respect to our ability to manage stress. When this spiritual component is also incorporated into this level of the cognitive filter, we have erected a basic framework to support the means by which we will navigate through life and, by implication, deal with stress.

All of these initial inputs to our cognitive filter have a direct and profound impact upon the physiological, psychological and spiritual expressions of our being that are presented to the world. These manifest in the genetic attributes, tendencies and predispositions we express as the components of who we are. Much has been made recently of the importance of genetic predisposition to certain diseases, but predisposition goes much further than that. It also encompasses our totality of personal preferences, behavioral tendencies, and basic personality strengths and weaknesses. This framework is initially filled in with the components of our own biomechanical individuality, toxicity levels, nutritional status, and endocrine balance. Let's look at each of these in turn.

Each of us has a distinct gait, a way of posturing ourselves in different situations, and using certain portions of our anatomy. These biomechanical habits are generated as a function of the previously mentioned influences. Here's a personal example: When I stand erect, I have a tendency to let my left foot toe out somewhat. I have worked with several chiropractors, body workers, Rolfers, massage therapists, personal trainers, etc. to attempt to correct this apparent misalignment. However, I've been told by more than one of them that this is most likely a function of previous injuries, the muscle and skeletal structure I was endowed with at birth, and the patterns of use that have dominated the way I stand and walk over the course of my life. That is biomechanical individuality.

Additionally, because of the unique environmental factors we each have been exposed to, the level and mix of different chemical and biological toxins in each of us is also unique. Again using a personal example, I grew up in the household of a smoker, long before the current level of awareness concerning secondhand smoke. As such, I have a predisposition toward developing certain types of lung ailments; many of us share this predisposition.

Further, our individual nutritional likes and dislikes, as well as the availability or lack of certain foods in our environment create both the fills and gaps in our nutritional status. In effect, this means that what you eat (or don't eat) has a profound effect on how you think. There are many foods that exert such effects on our thought processes, but none have a greater effect than our old nemesis caffeine. How many people do you know who, after a cup of strong coffee or a large caffeinated cola, are 'wired' for hours thereafter? I rest my case.

All of these factors exert a direct and profound effect on the balance or imbalance which manifests in our endocrine, or glandular, system, the primary manager and balancer of our body's available energy. We will devote an entire chapter to this subject later in the book.

A further filling in of our cognitive filter occurs with our unique psychological features, personality, emotional and behavioral characteristics. Some of these are learned from our primary caregivers while we are growing up, some from our peers, some are inherited genetically, and some are directed and shaped by our life experiences. Additionally, our social support system (or lack thereof), coping abilities, and degree of general 'hardiness' help also to fill in the factors that comprise our cognitive filter. All contribute to the way we view our world and, therefore, to our current state of health and the way we handle stress.

There are three important additional ideas that require discussion to reach a complete understanding of the cognitive filter. The first is that *the cognitive filter is constantly changing.* Every life experience we undergo, positive or negative, contributes to the structure of the cognitive filter. It operates on the principle of a feedback loop: events occur which we interpret and digest mentally (and therefore physically), and these interpretations either reinforce or negate our perceptions of ourselves, other people, and events taking place around us, thus altering the cognitive filter as it encounters the next event. In other words, our perceptions and our reaction to them continually shape our reality! This is especially important to understand when we deal with stress.

Second, it is equally important to remember that *the combination of stressors varies with each individual*, and that *each person responds differently to stress*. As mentioned earlier, since the mid-1950s the scientific community has accepted the fact that we are biochemically unique and respond differently to biochemical influences than the next person. We can now expand that definition and state that, through the influence of the cognitive filter, we also are unique in our ability to respond to stress.

As we have seen, there are a large number of variables which impact our cognitive filter. Each of these variables has a different impact on each of us. Some people have the ability to withstand enormous amounts of stress for extended periods without noticeable ill effect. Others seem to fall apart at the drop of a hat. The difference between the two is not only the coping ability of the person, but the difference in the relative influence and magnitude of all the factors which impact each person's ability to handle stress.

The third factor, and perhaps the most important to understand, is that *the impact of all these influences on our stress load is cumulative.* Whether we look at the positive or negative aspects of our cognitive filter, each aspect, to the extent it is reinforced and repeated, exerts a cumulative effect on how we view the world and, by implication, how we handle stress. In other words, add the effects of each of the scenarios I discussed, and others much like them, many times over, in many different contexts, each time they occur in our lives. It's when these conflicting needs, experiences and expectations brush against each other, again and again, like pieces of sandpaper rubbing together, that we experience stress. This cumulative aspect will be discussed in detail in a later chapter.

When we add the influence of the cognitive filter to our Stress Stack, it grows to three blocks, looking like this:

Dietary Influences (Foods and Beverages Which Cause Stress)	Caffeine, Artificial Sweeteners, Processed Sugar, White Flour, Trans Fats
Lifestyle Influences (Activities and Habits Which Cause Stress)	Driving in Traffic, Inactivity, Sleep Deprivation, Relationships
The "Cognitive Filter" (The Prism Through Which We View the World)	Physical, Mental, Emotional and Spiritual Inputs

The Fourth Block: The Nutritional Gap. This part of the Stress Stack refers to the difference between what your body requires nutritionally to adequately support a healthful stress response, and what it actually receives on a daily basis. One of the prevalent myths surrounding the science of nutrition, and promoted for years by the medical and dietetics communities, is the adage of "*eat a balanced diet and you don't need to take vitamins.*" While this would be true in an ideal situation, none of us live in that ideal situation. The legitimacy of this adage is compromised by several very important factors.

The first is contained in the very words of the adage. "*Eat a balanced diet,*" by definition, means selecting from a wide variety of ALL foods so we may obtain all the vitamins, minerals, and other nutrients necessary to sustain a healthy body. Unfortunately, published surveys show that the percentage of the population that truly eats a balanced diet varies between less than 1 per cent, and up to 20 per cent. These statistics should be questioned, because they rely on consumer self-reporting as a primary method of data gathering; it is very likely that the actual numbers are lower. So with all due respect to the well-meaning advice of the medical community, and assuming that the above data is truly accurate, that means that between 80 and 99 per cent of the American population blatantly ignore their advice.

Give this data, why do the medical and dietetics communities persist in reciting this obviously outmoded mantra, and do so in such strongly worded terms?

A primary part of the answer for the medical community can be found in a 1998 article in the *Archives of Internal Medicine*, the research publishing arm of the *Journal of the American Medical Association* (JAMA), where two courageous doctors revealed the hollowness of the medical community's objections to the use of nutritional supplements, a primary means that over half the American public uses to fill in the gaps of their diets.

Titled *Battling Quackery*, the article itself is only four pages long with heavy footnoting, but contains much wisdom evident even to the layperson. Briefly, the authors cite the combination of uncritical acceptance of news of supplement toxicity (even if poorly documented), shoddy scholarship on the subject of supplements in medical textbooks, and stubborn, almost contrarian, rejection of hard evidence of effectiveness as indicative of the medical community's institutional bias against use of nutritional supplements.

But perhaps the authors' most convincing argument was :

"Part of the resistance stems from the fact that the potential benefits of micronutrients were advanced by outsiders (i.e., not of the medical community; author's italics added), who took their message directly to the public, and part from the fact that the concept of a deficiency disease did not fit well with prevailing biomedical paradigms, particularly the germ theory."

In other words, if you're not a member of 'the club,' and you don't talk the party line, you're not qualified to talk about the subject of health at all.

On the other hand, the position of the dietetics community, represented primarily by the American Dietetic Association (ADA; and now known as the Academy of Nutrition and Dietetics (AND)), is a prime example of the inappropriate role of what I call 'advocacy science' in the creation and dissemination of information to the public on proper diet, nutrition and lifestyle. From sources as diverse as JAMA, Discover magazine, and the Life Extension Foundation, the alarm is being sounded concerning the influence of 'advocacy science,' i.e., science pursued strictly to advance financial gain. This type of scientific inquiry has its genesis in a little known but very important piece of legislation passed over 30 years ago.

In 1965, prior to enactment of the legislation, 60 per cent of US scientific research was conducted in government laboratories. By 2006, 65 per cent was conducted by private companies. The primary impetus to this change was enactment of the 1980 University and Small Business Patent Procedures Act (P.L. 96-517, Patent and Trademark Act Amendments of 1980) otherwise known as the Bayh-Dole Act. By lifting the restrictions on researchers owning and profiting from their discoveries, it was hoped that the resulting greater and more varied research would stimulate wider advances in every field of science. Coupled with the closure of many government laboratories as a cost-cutting measure during the Reagan administration, it resulted in a wholesale redirection of scientific research from the public to the private sector.

Although in some respects the intent of Bayh-Dole has been fulfilled, an unintended consequence has been the development of a culture of 'science for sale.' Now, in virtually every field of science, and especially in health care, research consultants can parlay the 'halo effect' of their advanced academic credentials to lend credence before the public to their corporate sponsors' claims concerning the sponsors' products and services.

Conversely, these same consultants can be employed to structure research which questions the effectiveness of a competitor's products and services. This is a prevalent use of 'advocacy science' in the health care system, especially by pharmaceutical companies who wish to discredit a particular natural product or service.

Also, there exist no uniform standards, inside the government or out, to require disclosure of the financial ties between a health care researcher and the company underwriting his/her research. Numerous examples exist of studies published in peer-reviewed journals where this information was deliberately omitted. The scale of this problem was the genesis of the critical 2006 JAMA article *The Influence of Money on Medical Science,* written by Catherine deAngelis, then the JAMA editor-in-chief.

The practical result has been that the body of scientific knowledge surrounding diet and nutrition is heavily skewed by the financial interests of the major food industries and processed food manufacturers. This is evident, first, from the composition of the USDA *Food Pyramid* (now known as the *Food Plate*) and, second, from the sources of financial support offered the ADN and its state affiliates.

The financial connections between the AND, its state affiliates, and the major processed food companies are clearly displayed on the AND web site (http://www.eatright.org/corporatesponsors). The AND's listing, with effusive thanks, of Aramark®, The Coca Cola Company®, The National Dairy Council®, Pepsico®, Unilever®, Abbott Nutrition®, Cargill (Corowise®), General Mills®, Kellogg's®, Mars® Incorporated, Hershey®, McNeil Nutritionals® LLC (Johnson & Johnson®), Truvia®, and SoyJoy® (Pharmavite® LLC) (several of whose products are displayed in the American family picture later in this chapter), clearly demonstrates their organization's indebtedness to these companies. The obligation of the AND to provide unbiased, objective nutritional advice to the American public is thus compromised by the conflicting obligation to assist their benefactors in advancing their collective commercial interests.

Predictably, the AND vehemently denies that this financial support has any effect on the objectivity of their advice. In fact, in a hearing on their (unsuccessful) exclusionary licensing bill during the 2009 Texas legislative session, one dietitian flatly denied that they even received financial support at all!

Ironically, compelling evidence to the contrary appeared in one of the very sources the AND and the AMA both cite most for support of their own position. A 2006 JAMA article titled *Health Industry Practices That Create Conflicts of Interest*, authored by a distinguished group of MD and PhD researchers, debunked the myth that gifting at any level did not have an impact. Specifically, the paper said:

"Social science research demonstrates that the impulse to reciprocate for even small gifts is a powerful influence on people's behavior. Individuals receiving gifts are often unable to remain objective; they reweigh information and choices in light of the gift."

Equally important was the authors' assessment of the effect of financially influenced advice on patient care:

"[A] systematic review of the medical literature on gifting. . . found that an overwhelming majority of interactions had negative results on clinical care."

Interestingly, resistance to this inappropriate relationship has already sprung up, from not only within the health care practitioner community, but also from the US Congress. A group of concerned physicians, nutritionists and dietitians have formed ReallyEatRight.org as a means of educating the public about what's really going on inside the AND. Additionally, US Senator Charles Grassley has launched an investigation into the relationship between the AND and their sponsors, demanding full disclosure of their financial ties. As of this writing, the AND has disclosed that they have received over $1 million from pharmaceutical companies, but have so far refused to reveal the extent of their financial ties to major food companies.

Likewise, it is apparent that, in the development of the *Food Plate,* the USDA also was and is unduly influenced by political pressure exerted by food production associations. Some of the recommended portion sizes are up to eight times the size of portions recommended in other countries, although the number of portions recommended are the same.

Dan Glickman, Agricultural Secretary from 1995 through 2001, tacitly admitted as much:

"USDA basically was in an unusual role of not wanting to say that there were any good foods or any bad foods; that all foods were okay, [presumably] eaten in some degree of moderation or discretion. So USDA was always very careful at not defining evil as part of any particular food category."

Many nutrition experts characterize the problem in much blunter terms, asserting that the USDA has a conflict of interest between advancing the interests of the foods industry (by encouraging Americans to eat more food) and offering the American public nutritional guidelines that are so heavily influenced by that same industry. One of the most influential voices is Marion Nestle, professor of Nutrition, Food Studies, and Public Health at New York University, and author of the book *Food Politics:*

"We don't have an independent voice in the government advising the public about diet and health because if the government were to advise the public about diet and health, it would have to tell people to eat less junk food. And it can't do that... Because the companies that produce the junk food wouldn't stand for it."

In fact, when the USDA attempted to use the Food Pyramid to accurately portray the unhealthy effect of overconsumption of soft drinks, the beverage companies sued the government and, unfortunately, won.

The practical impact of these influences is clearly displayed by the food selection habits of Americans versus those in other nations.

Below are pictorial presentations of the weekly grocery purchases of an average American family versus one in Italy, a nation ranked #3 in Overall Health System Performance by the World Health Organization (WHO) in 1997:

Representative Weekly Diet of an American Family

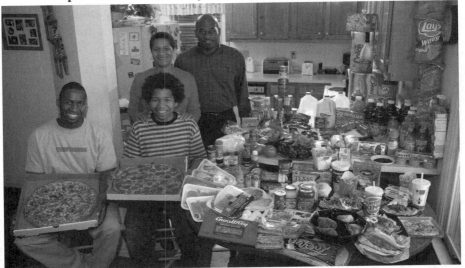

Representative Weekly Diet of an Italian Family

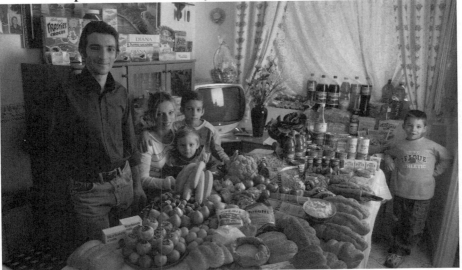

Photos by Menzel Photography. Provided by www.wie.org. Used by Permission

These data, and much more like them, conclusively demonstrate that the conventional health care system has failed the American public in effectively addressing the most serious threat to our nation's physical and fiscal health: the continued and growing prevalence of diet- and lifestyle-related illness in our society. At the same time, our government has permitted the major food production associations to exert an inappropriate level of influence on the public's education on the subject of nutrition, creating the situation graphically depicted by the contrasting photographs on the previous page, exacerbating the diet- and lifestyle-related challenges we face, and contributing substantively to the prevalence of chronic stress.

We have already discussed the second and third factors contributing to the nutritional gap: the fast food and high carbs that comprise the Standard American Diet, ironically abbreviated to SAD.

Additionally, our own personal food preferences contribute greatly to the problem. How many times have we heard someone say "*I don't like fish (or vegetables, or whatever nutritious food we may name)?*" If that person as a result deliberately avoids those types of foods, are they *truly* consuming a balanced diet?

Those who 'eat organic' may be smiling a self satisfied smile right now, convinced that they don't fall into that category. Not so fast! They, too, have food preferences, likes and dislikes, even if they are eating food that is demonstrably healthier. As such, they are *not* necessarily eating a balanced diet!

Finally, compelling evidence comes directly from the records of the US Department of Agriculture itself. In a study published in the *American Journal of Clinical Nutrition* in December 2004, a research team examined the change in nutrient content of common fruits and vegetables from 1950 through 1999. They found that the content had declined (depending on the produce and nutrient examined) between six and 38 per cent. This was attributed to the reduction in available soil nutrients that has occurred due to repeatedly growing the same crops on the same soil, as well as the use of fertilizers which support increased crop size and pleasing appearance but not increased nutrient value. In a nation with an obesity rate in excess of 60 per cent, the solution definitely is not to eat between six and 38 per cent more of these foods!

It is therefore safe to say that almost no one in America today eats a 'balanced diet,' and the gaps in the nutritional status of *all of us* contribute greatly to our ability or inability to handle stress. I can say with certainty that almost no one can do without nutritional supplementation, especially those nutrients which fuel our bodies' stress response. In other words, if you're not taking a good quality suite of nutritional supplements, you most likely are leaving your body's stress response mechanism open to exploitation by nutritional deficiencies. We will consider some of the effective alternatives to address these nutritional gaps in a later chapter.

Our Stress Stack continues to grow; we can now add the "Nutritional Gap" as a block of our stack:

Dietary Influences (Foods and Beverages Which Cause Stress)	Caffeine, Artificial Sweeteners, Processed Sugar, White Flour, Trans Fats
Lifestyle Influences (Activities and Habits Which Cause Stress)	Driving in Traffic, Inactivity, Sleep Deprivation, Relationships
The "Cognitive Filter" (The Prism Through Which We View the World)	Physical, Mental, Emotional and Spiritual Inputs
The Nutritional Gap (The Difference Between What Our Bodies Need and Get)	Social Conditioning, Personal Food Preferences, Gaps in Food Supply

The Fifth Block: Toxic Exposure. It is a little known fact that our species has been exposed to more chemicals and toxic influences in the last fifty years than during all the prior 200,000 years of human history combined. The US Environmental Protection Agency now requires safe handling notices to be posted in workplaces around the country for over a *half million chemicals!!!* The number of these toxins is increasing at the rate of about 5,000 annually.

While most of these chemicals have been developed for the purpose of enhancing our quality of life on this planet, there is definitely a down side. When these chemicals are disposed of, transported or mishandled, there is always a risk of toxic chemical exposure; these episodes are what we usually hear about in the media. However, it is the daily exposure we all undergo, in small increments, that holds the greatest potential for chronic stress and widespread ill health.

There have been many well-written books on the subject of toxic exposure, so I won't try to duplicate their efforts here. However, the best one I have seen, from a self-help standpoint, is *The Detox Solution*, by my colleague Dr. Patricia Fitzgerald. She has appeared on TV and radio to discuss her findings, and they are worth reading in her own words. See the Resources section for how to obtain this important and helpful book.

There is no doubt that the fertilizers and pesticides which are used to help grow our crops of fruits and vegetables are valuable aids to the productivity of American farmers. The 'Breadbasket of America' is truly a success story. But as time has gone on, we have discovered that this unbridled productivity has a definite down side. The chemicals we have used on our fruits and vegetables did not increase the nutritional value of the food, but were used to grow bigger, better looking crops that sell well at the market. In the process (as mentioned in the previous section), we have progressively grown less and less nutritious food, and paid the additional price of chronically exposing ourselves to continuing doses of these same chemicals.

When we look across the huge spectrum of products which have been created over the last century to help make our lives easier, there is a common denominator for many of them: they are made of synthetic chemicals derived from petroleum. While these plastics, cleaners, machine parts, etc. all serve productive functions, many of them also have an unintended side effect: when introduced into the body, even in small doses, they mimic the effects of certain hormones, especially estrogen. As such, they have been collectively assigned the name xenoestrogens ('xeno' being a prefix meaning "*from a foreign source*"). The impact of these substances is that, once they are introduced into the body, they migrate to the same receptor sites on our cells as do the real estrogens produced by our own hormonal systems. Once there, they act as a multiplier of the effects of real estrogen, including the tissue proliferation associated with uterine, breast, and other forms of cancer.

How do they get there? Let's look at a couple of examples. Many if not most of us have purchased and consumed bottled water at one time or another. If we were to look at the bottom of that bottle (regardless of the brand), we would see the number '1' in the triangular recycling symbol. That indicates, among other things, that the plastic used to manufacture that bottle is the softest, cheapest type available for that purpose. As such, it is very susceptible to changes in temperature, such that at high temperatures (like those sometimes encountered during long distance shipping), molecules of the plastic actually slough off into the water, which we then consume.

Each time this occurs it creates a small amount of stress; the human body is easily able to handle this negligible individual load. But if it is a recurring pattern, and is reinforced by other activities such as heating or microwaving food in similar soft plastic containers, these chemicals can, over time, build up in the human body to toxic levels, accentuating the effects of hormones like estrogen and making the likelihood of the occurrence of serious illnesses such as cancer much greater.

A second source of these xenoestrogens is found in the chemicals used to process and manufacture cosmetics products. Many of the ingredients in these products, designed to sooth and beautify the skin, have the unintended consequence of adding to the xenoestrogenic load and again increasing the likelihood of serious illness. All of that, collectively and cumulatively, is stress.

Another category of toxic exposure is prescription drugs. The natural and alternative health community has a *major* disagreement with the medical and pharmaceutical communities concerning the use of synthetic versus natural substances for therapeutic purposes. The medical community asserts (and quite a few of their studies show) that a synthetic source of a chemical is equally safe and effective as a natural source.

However, their argument begins to break down when the subject of drug side effects is addressed. All substances introduced into the human body, whether they are natural or synthetic, derive their mechanism of action from interacting with (latching onto, really) the cell receptor sites having to do with the particular physiological activity the substance addresses.

In the case of natural substances, innumerable studies have shown conclusively that natural substances interact completely with the appropriate cell receptor sites. Not so with synthetic substances. Even if the chemical composition is identical to a natural substance, the mechanism of action is not quite as effective as it is with the natural substance.

This is the comprehensive explanation for why synthetic prescription drugs generate side effects. When the synthetic molecular structure of the drug does not align accurately with the cell receptor site, side effects result. These side effects cause stress. Combine that with the fact that many of our prescription drugs are also combined with stress-causing ingredients like caffeine, and we have a real 'witches' brew' of stress generating ingredients.

For all these reasons, toxic influences can also be added to our Stress Stack:

Dietary Influences (Foods and Beverages Which Cause Stress)	Caffeine, Artificial Sweeteners, Processed Sugar, White Flour, Trans Fats
Lifestyle Influences (Activities and Habits Which Cause Stress)	Driving in Traffic, Inactivity, Sleep Deprivation, Relationships
The "Cognitive Filter" (The Prism Through Which We View the World)	Physical, Mental, Emotional and Spiritual Inputs
The Nutritional Gap (The Difference Between What Our Bodies Need and Get)	Social Conditioning, Personal Food Preferences, Gaps in Food Supply
Toxic Influences (External Chemical, Biological or Radiological Stressors)	Xenoestrogens, Prescription Drugs, EMF, Chemicals, Fungi/ Bacteria

The Sixth Block: The Trigger Factor. Many people know one or more persons they can describe like this: they have appeared to be in good health for many years. However, when they experience a traumatic event in their lives, such as the loss of a spouse or child, a job loss, or another traumatic event such as an injury-causing accident, they are never the same, healthwise, again. Their health starts a long downward slide (sometimes slow, sometimes fast) that frequently results in either permanent disability or premature death.

Do *you* know anyone like that? Or worse yet, are you one of these people? What causes these healthy-appearing people to undergo this unpleasant experience? I call it the 'trigger factor,' the straw that breaks the camel's back.

Because most people think linearly about their health, they assume that this single incident is responsible for their descent into ill health. In most cases, however, this event simply pushes their bodies over the edge, as opposed to being the proximate cause of ill health. When their stress loads are examined more closely, it becomes apparent that they quite frequently have been carrying a very high stress burden for a very long period of time. The combination of their dietary influences, lifestyle influences, the operation of their cognitive filter, their nutritional gap and their toxic burden have teetered for years on the brink of ill health. In reality, it is the accumulation of the other five Stress Stack factors' influences, combined with the 'trigger,' that overwhelms the body's ability to respond.

As such, we can now add the 'trigger factor' to our individual Stress Stack:

Dietary Influences (Foods and Beverages Which Cause Stress)	Caffeine, Artificial Sweeteners, Processed Sugar, White Flour, Trans Fats
Lifestyle Influences (Activities and Habits Which Cause Stress)	Driving in Traffic, Inactivity, Sleep Deprivation, Relationships
The "Cognitive Filter" (The Prism Through Which We View the World)	Physical, Mental, Emotional and Spiritual Inputs
The Nutritional Gap (The Difference Between What Our Bodies Need and Get)	Social Conditioning, Personal Food Preferences, Gaps in Food Supply
Toxic Influences (External Chemical, Biological or Radiological Stressors)	Xenoestrogens, Prescription Drugs, EMF, Chemicals, Fungi/ Bacteria
Trigger Factor	Job Loss, Death of a Spouse/Child, Automobile Accident, etc.

The Catabolic Threshold: The Definition of 'The Brink.' In our discussion of the 'trigger factor,' we talked about how the combination of stressors can push our body over the edge into ill health.
But what exactly is the edge, the brink?

When you analyze the processes at work in the human body, they can be broken down into two major categories: anabolic (Webster: the constructive part of metabolism concerned especially with macromolecular synthesis) or catabolic (Webster: destructive metabolism involving the release of energy and resulting in the breakdown of complex materials within the organism).

The human body is a marvelous adaptive mechanism. It can compensate for large amounts of change in the body and, therefore, deal with large amounts of stress. However, as we will see in an upcoming chapter, every one of us has a finite energy bank available to fuel this compensating mechanism. When we exhaust this energy bank, we push our bodies beyond the point at which they can continue to function normally. It is this point, this threshold, which defines the border between health and disease. Therefore, the border can be accurately defined as the 'catabolic threshold.'

It is important to note that this threshold is dynamic. It is affected by both the mix and magnitude of the other parts of the Stress Stack. The larger and more influential the other parts are, the closer the body moves toward the catabolic threshold. The smaller they are, the further away the threshold moves. Here's a visual comparison of these two states:

Stress Stack of a Healthy Individual
Catabolic Threshold

Dietary Influences (Foods and Beverages Which Cause Stress)	Caffeine, Artificial Sweeteners, Processed Sugar, White Flour, Trans Fats
Lifestyle Influences (Activities and Habits Which Cause Stress)	Driving in Traffic, Inactivity, Sleep Deprivation, Relationships
The "Cognitive Filter" (The Prism Through Which We View the World)	Physical, Mental, Emotional and Spiritual Inputs
The Nutritional Gap (The Difference Between What Our Bodies Need and Get)	Social Conditioning, Personal Food Preferences, Gaps in Food Supply
Toxic Influences (External Chemical, Biological or Radiological Stressors)	Xenoestrogens, Prescription Drugs, EMF, Chemicals, Fungi/ Bacteria
Trigger Factor	Job Loss, Death of a Spouse/Child, Automobile Accident, etc.

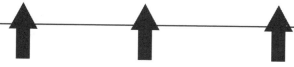

Stress Stack of an Individual in Ill Health
Catabolic Threshold

Dietary Influences (Foods and Beverages Which Cause Stress)	Caffeine, Artificial Sweeteners, Processed Sugar, White Flour, Trans Fats
Lifestyle Influences (Activities and Habits Which Cause Stress)	Driving in Traffic, Inactivity, Sleep Deprivation, Relationships
The "Cognitive Filter" (The Prism Through Which We View the World)	Physical, Mental, Emotional and Spiritual Inputs
The Nutritional Gap (The Difference Between What Our Bodies Need and Get)	Social Conditioning, Personal Food Preferences, Gaps in Food Supply
Toxic Influences (External Chemical, Biological or Radiological Stressors)	Xenoestrogens, Prescription Drugs, EMF, Chemicals, Fungi/ Bacteria
Trigger Factor	Job Loss, Death of a Spouse/Child, Automobile Accident, etc.

The significance of the catabolic threshold cannot be overstated. Once the human body crosses this threshold, the focus of health care switches from health maintenance to health restoration. We abruptly transition from preventing disease to conquering it. Depending on the composition of the individual's Stress Stack, this transition can be either relatively brief, or long, arduous and frequently painful.

In summary, the Stress Stack is a descriptive model that allows each of us to better understand all of the unique, dynamic, cumulative and holistic characteristics of our personal set of stressors. As the ensuing chapters will demonstrate, it also gives us a clearer idea of which stressors we can control and change, and which ones we must compensate for. Finally, the Stress Stack offers a way for us to qualitatively gage how close each of us are to crossing the catabolic threshold.

So far, we've looked at what stress is and how it can be described by our Stress Stack. But exactly what factors in our society and our daily lives cause our bodies to actually get from Point A (good health) to Point B (crossing the catabolic threshold into illness)? In order to answer that, we must examine the complex interplay of societal, governmental, health care and individual behavioral factors that exert a direct impact on the activation of our stress response. Turn the page to continue empowering yourself.

CHAPTER 2

AMERICA'S SELF-INFLICTED WOUND:
STRESS, PRODUCTIVITY AND THE HEALTH CARE CRISIS

"Discontent is the first step in the progress of a man or a nation."

— Oscar Wilde

Given the myriad stressors which impact American society today, it is of utmost importance that individuals and organizations alike come to a more complete understanding of stress if they are to take meaningful action to alleviate its effects.

How pervasive is this problem? It is estimated that one hundred years ago the average American took in about 600 impressions a day that caused action or reaction in thought or deed. However, Wayne Dyer, PhD cites research showing that today that number is *60,000* a day! In other words, within a single century we have experienced a hundredfold increase in the number of events with which we must contend on a daily basis, and which, individually and collectively, have the potential to cause stress.

In their book *The Stress Solution*, Lyle H. Miller, PhD, and Alma Dell Smith, PhD estimate that 75 per cent to 90 per cent of visits to family physicians are for complaints/illnesses whose root cause is stress. According to Prof. Melissa Chessher of Syracuse University, stress accounts for 70 to 90 per cent of corporate employee hospital visits.

Stress-related ill health is not cheap. The American Institute of Stress (AIS) estimates that stress related ailments cost US companies about $300 billion a year in absenteeism, being late to work, reduced productivity, and the loss of valuable employees. More than half of employees (55 per cent) surveyed by the American Psychological Association in 2007 said they were less productive at work as a result of stress. The costs are also reflected in the fact that 4 out of 10 corporate 'sick outs' are stress related. Said another way, workplace stress causes approximately one million US employees to miss work each day!

One would think that, confronted with such a pervasive problem, our nation would act decisively to mobilize whatever resources are required to solve it. Yet the reality is that our collective response has been disjointed, fraught with parochial influences, and largely ineffective. Why is that? The answer lies in understanding the influence of our societal structure on the problem, as well as that of our government and our business community.

Setting the Stage: The Societal Framework. When examining our society at its most basic level, it is readily apparent that we are a sub optimizing society. The Webster dictionary defines the words *sub optimize* to mean "*with repetition (as of a process) so as to form, stress, or deal with subordinate parts or relations.*" Applied to a societal structure like ours, it means that we all belong to one or more groups, units or organizations which are focused on making their little piece of the puzzle as perfect as possible. Oftentimes this is done without regard to, or perhaps in direct conflict with, the needs and desires of the units and organizations around and above them.

Another description for this behavior is *tribalism* (Webster: tribal consciousness and loyalty; especially: exaltation of the tribe above other groups). Whether we are talking about our family, our school, our professional organization, our company, or our country, our society is structured to promote and reward behavior that benefits the particular 'tribe' (group, unit or organization) we are a part of over the needs and interests of the other groups we belong to.

There is some fascinating, preliminary, ongoing research in the field of sociobiology whose results contend that tribal behavior is a genetically inherited trait; however, conclusive evidence of the validity of this theory as applied to humans has yet to be provided. Regardless, if we look closely we clearly see a large body of evidence around us that supports this contention.

To an extent perhaps unmatched in our country's history, the business, political, religious, and cultural components of our society are all wracked by varying degrees of conflict among the various 'tribes' that comprise these communities. These same communities are simultaneously interacting contentiously with each other. Some prominent examples include the conflict between the climatological portion of the scientific community with the energy industry, and the decades-long conflict between the 'pro life' and 'pro choice' factions of contemporary culture.

A compelling argument can indeed be made that the larger a given group to which we belong becomes, the less homogeneous it becomes, and therefore the more challenging it is to obtain consensus from the group as to what behaviors are beneficial to that group. The outcomes of the national elections of 2000 through 2010 are perfect examples, but we can also see this displayed at smaller organizational levels.

For example, prior to moving to Austin, my wife and I lived in a small city in south central Texas which, like many around us, has rapidly grown from a sleepy, slow moving rural community to a true suburb of the much larger San Antonio to its southeast. In fact, during the year 2008, the city was identified as one of the fastest growing in the nation.

When we first moved there in 2004, and prior to the onset of this rapid growth, it was a small, relatively homogenous city, with a cadre of dedicated citizen volunteers who conscientiously maintained the years-long status quo of a friendly, collegial place to live, with a 'small town,' rural atmosphere. It prided itself as being able to maintain that small town, country atmosphere despite the rapid growth of the communities around it.

However, the town eventually became caught up in that growth as well, in the space of four years almost tripling in population. This irrevocably shifted the demographics to favor the segment of the populace which supported increased city services, as well as increased expenditures for those services.

Many of these people had moved there from much larger communities, where ready access to extensive city and business services was available. While they greatly appreciated the small town atmosphere, they did not want to have to drive long distances to, for example, shop for groceries, buy a Starbucks®, or eat at a nice restaurant. The resultant conflict between these citizens, and those who favored slower or no growth, set the stage for continued gridlock on the city council, and creation of a poisonous political atmosphere where little was accomplished.

The same process is at work when any company or other organization interfaces with societal entities larger than itself (e.g., the local, state or national government). In this case the interactions are far more complex, and involve far larger and more diverse groups of people. I have extensive personal experience with such situations as a result of both my military leadership and political advocacy activities.

In the military arena, in 1990-1991, I served as the operations officer (second in command) for the 325th Bomb Squadron at Fairchild Air Force Base, near Spokane, Washington. The 325th was at that time the largest B-52 bomber squadron in the Air Force's Strategic Air Command (SAC), with over 160 assigned crewmembers of six different crew specialties, comprising 27 six man B-52 flight crews. During my tenure as operations officer, the squadron had successfully navigated a number of challenges: earning an 'outstanding' rating from a rigorous operational readiness inspection; deploying crews and airplanes to Diego Garcia, Australia and Korea; and sending six hand-picked crews in theater to augment the B-52 units deployed to support Operation Desert Storm. As a result, by the summer of 1991 the morale of the squadron was very high. We were all looking forward to the challenges of the future.

Then, in August 1991, the Soviet Union fell. Virtually overnight, everything in the B-52 world changed. There was now no longer a need for the constant, hair-trigger, nuclear alert posture for one third of the B-52 bomber fleet, a posture that had been maintained since the 1950s. I was honored to be present on the alert ramp the day all of our squadron's alert bombers were taken off alert. For someone who had spent over half their 20 year Air Force career in the alert business, it was a deeply moving experience to see the fruits of one's labor come to a successful conclusion. The US had won the Cold War, and the world was able to take a giant step back from the nuclear abyss. I took great pride in shaking the hands of each crewmember that day, thanking them for a job that was truly and completely well done.

Shortly afterward, I was transferred to the new operations support squadron (OSS), comprising the over 200 staff members in the bomber wing who supported the flying operation. I served there first as the operations officer, helping to get the new unit organized and running, and then briefly as commander before I retired from the military in mid-1992. During that period, I saw first hand the effects of further, profound change being implemented at both the national and local level.

SAC, long the backbone of our country's defense establishment, was no longer needed and was scheduled for dissolution on June 1, 1992. Its remaining airplanes and crew assets were being transferred to a newly established Air Combat Command. Entire B-52 units were slated for early closure, the airplanes to be decommissioned and either destroyed or sent to long-term storage.

Simultaneously, the Air Force announced the beginning of a reduction in force, or RIF. Crew positions such as B-52 electronic warfare officer and gunner, once considered secure career paths, were now vastly overmanned. Screening boards would convene to select only 10 per cent of junior officers in select aircrew specialties for retention. The remaining 90 per cent of the junior officers in the career field would be involuntarily separated or, in the case of the enlisted aerial gunner specialty, retrained and reassigned.

The Air Force did attempt to entice crew members to voluntarily separate, offering them a bonus to do so before the RIF board convened. As OSS commander, it was my task to counsel each of the members of my squadron whom the RIF boards would impact, and give them my perspective on their chances of surviving a RIF. It was a portion of my job I did not relish. Day after day, I spent countless hours in face-to-face counseling sessions with bright, motivated young aircrew members, most of them still wanting to continue their Air Force careers, but facing an almost zero chance of being able to do so. The stress these young people had to contend with, making life changing decisions almost on the spot, is a prime example of what occurs when a large organization undergoes profound change. In this case, I saw firsthand how the needs of the larger organization (i.e., the Air Force's need to re-size its officer and enlisted corps in the face of rapidly changing circumstances) directly conflicted with not only the needs of its smaller units (i.e., the need for the squadron to maintain adequate manning and member morale) but also those of the members themselves (i.e., the need for job security).

I have similar experience in the political advocacy arena. In late 2006, I became a founding member of an organization called the Texas Health Freedom Coalition (THFC). Our group was formed to allow the Texas natural health community to have a greater voice at the Texas state legislature. At that time, the Texas natural health community was very fragmented, its diverse groups pursuing generally similar goals but in a totally uncoordinated fashion. As such, we could neither mount a coordinated defense against professional incursions by competing groups, such as the state medical association or dietetics association, nor pursue our own positive goals, such as enacting health freedom legislation. Thanks primarily to the efforts of my friend and colleague, attorney Rick Jaffe, we convened a statewide conference of all the 'chiefs' in November 2006. Thus was the THFC born. Partly as a function of my prior leadership and organizational experience, my fellow executive committee members asked me to chair the THFC, a position I have held for over five years. I am honored at their continued confidence in me.

The two primary management challenges I have faced in this capacity are to help shape the working relationship among the disparate 16 original groups (later expanded to 20) into a cohesive whole, and to work with my fellow committee members to craft the strategy we would use when interacting with the Texas state legislature and the executive branch of the state government. Each of these groups has their own agenda, and each addresses the issues we all have an interest in from their own point of view. Many times, discussion of these issues has resulted in either internal disagreement (among the THFC member organizations), or disagreement between the THFC and the various state governmental bodies. Any of these situations causes some degree of stress for the members of the groups involved.

Additionally, an important part of my postgraduate education, which includes a masters degree in management and supervision, was the study of organizational behavior and change. Some of you may recall that one of the original definitions of stress is "*the non-specific response of the body to any demand for change.*" If we apply that definition to organizational settings like the ones above, we can clearly see that the same process is at work in organizations which undergo any kind of change and, therefore, experience stress as a result of that change. Best-selling books such as *Who Moved My Cheese?* have brought this issue into the public spotlight, and highlight the complex and dynamic characteristics of any organization undergoing substantive change. Because success in adapting to change is so crucial to dealing effectively with chronic stress, Chapter 7 of this book is devoted entirely to the subject.

If we were to try to quantitatively describe the myriad interactions that occur among groups such as those described above, we would be delving into some of the most complex and arcane areas of mathematics, such as differential calculus. Most people, me included, do not possess the training or skill to understand or manipulate such complex analytical tools. Suffice it to say that the interactions between and among these 'tribes' affect countless people in ways many of them don't even comprehend. However, it is clear that, to the extent that these interactions create differences of opinion or conflict, they also create stress.

9/11 and America's Stress: Taking it to a Whole New Level. Every society throughout history experiences events which define their character and shape the way they operate. In the preface to this book, I alluded to an event that virtually every member of the 'Baby Boom' generation vividly recalls: the landing of the first man on the moon. Were you to ask any Baby Boomer where s/he was on that day, chances are they would be able to recall with great detail. It was one of those historical experiences that almost everyone wanted to be a part of, even if vicariously.

Unfortunately, those are not the only events that people vividly recall. Ask any member of my parents' generation, and they will easily recall where they were and what they were doing on December 7, 1941, the day the Japanese bombed Pearl Harbor and triggered our participation in World War II. The same applies to the events of September 11, 2001. If you are reading these words, you undoubtedly know where you were, whom you were with, and what you were doing on that tragic day. And like the rest of us, you have experienced firsthand the consequences of that day, and the increase in chronic stress that resulted.

The first imposition of that stress took place on the actual day itself, and continued for weeks thereafter. In contrast to the dissemination of the news about Pearl Harbor, which occurred primarily by a combination of word of mouth, newspapers and radio (and only later via newsreel footage in the movie theaters of that time), the entire story of the destruction of the World Trade Center, the attack on the Pentagon, and the events occurring on Flight 93 were brought to us instantaneously and in excruciating detail via worldwide television. Over the next days and weeks, we were subjected to constant repetition of those images, which are now burned into the collective psyche of both the nation and the entire world, and have contributed directly to the collective increase in our stress level.

The consequences of those events have also added other components to our collective stress. For example, we now live under a 'threat advisory system,' which replaced the original color coded system implemented immediately after 9/11. Although not as intrusive or alarmist as the color coded system, the overarching existence and influence of the threat advisory system nevertheless serves as a constant reminder that our society is not as safe as it once was.

Additionally, the post-9/11 passage and implementation of the *Patriot Act*, which put into place a demonstrable contraction of our personal freedoms in favor of personal and societal safety, contributes directly to the climate of constant, almost daily, reminder of our degraded safety and, correspondingly, our increased stress.

Prior to that day, consumer interaction with the airline industry, though already changed considerably by deregulation, was still a relatively benign experience. A trip to an airline terminal, though sometimes crowded, was at least seen as relatively safe.

9/11 changed all that. As a former airline captain, I recall vividly the weeks after, when nearly empty planes, populated by fearful passengers and crews, attempted to get the airline industry's legs under it again. It took a lot of TLC by the crews of all the airline carriers, offered day-by-day and passenger-by-passenger, to bring the public's trust back up to where it is today. Hats off to all of my fellow crewmembers who helped facilitate that shift in public perception.

At the same time, 9/11 has forever and fundamentally altered the airline passenger experience. When you examine the process a typical passenger undergoes from the time s/he enters an airline terminal until they board the aircraft, it can only be characterized as a gradual but inexorable ceding of control over one's person. The combination of the baggage check, passenger screening, and accompanying control mechanisms (i.e., passenger queues at security checkpoints, whole body scanners, the substantial presence of Transportation Security Administration (TSA) personnel, etc.) have created a much more tightly controlled environment, and one which is generally perceived as more stressful by the traveling passenger. I know of many people who, faced with the prospect of such an environment, have chosen to drive to their destinations instead of fly. The effect on the financial condition of the airline industry has not been positive, and the resulting large scale displacement of laid-off airline employees only adds to our nation's collective stress.

This is in spite of the fact that an analysis conducted by the University of Michigan showed that over a thousand more people died on the roads in the United States in the first three months after 9/11 than would have been expected for that time period, reinforcing the conclusion that, despite the prevailing public perception, flying remains a much safer activity than driving.

How significant is this cumulative, societal stress? University of California Irvine researchers E.A. Holman, R.C. Silver and their colleagues conducted a 3-year study which examined the experience of over 2,700 Americans to determine what effect, if any, the events of 9/11 contributed to changes in their state of health. The study found that "*acute stress responses to the 9/11 attacks were associated with a 53 per cent increased incidence of cardiovascular ailments over the 3 subsequent years, even after adjusting for pre-9/11 cardiovascular and mental health status, degree of exposure to the attacks, (and other risk factors).*"

A later follow-up study, also conducted by Holman and Silver, found, "*after the collective stress of 9/11, rates of physical ailments...including cardiovascular, endocrine, gastrointestinal, and hematology-oncology ailments (cancer) increased.*" "*... doctor-diagnosed illness climbed by 18 per cent in a nationally representative sample of adults.*"

Additionally, scientists at Mount Sinai School of Medicine and the University of Edinburgh studied the relationship between maternal PTSD symptoms and salivary cortisol levels in 38 women and their infants. Mothers who experienced symptoms of PTSD in response to 9/11 had lower cortisol levels compared to mothers who did not develop this condition, indicating an impaired ability to respond to stress.

Moreover, approximately one year after birth, the babies of those mothers had significantly lower cortisol levels compared to the babies of mothers who developed only minimal symptoms. This decrease in cortisol levels among the infants was similar to their mothers' hormonal response to PTSD, indicating the babies' decreased ability to respond to stress. I will discuss the relationship between cortisol and our ability to respond effectively to stress in a later chapter.

While these findings are admittedly preliminary, they comprise the compelling beginning of a body of work that demonstrates the correlation between first acute, then chronic stress, and ultimately the increased likelihood of the onset of serious illness.

All of this research also correlates with the preliminary conclusions reached by the National Institute on Drug Abuse, a division of the National Institutes of Health (NIH), which has stated:

"Research shows that Post Traumatic Stress Disorder (PTSD), a psychiatric disorder, may develop in people after they experience or witness life-threatening events such as terrorist incidents, military combat, natural disasters, serious accidents, or violent personal assaults like rape... Because the events that occurred on September 11, 2001, were experienced by thousands of people, as well as rescue workers in and around the vicinity of the attacks, and were televised to millions across the world, it is likely that some individuals may develop behavioral and emotional re-adjustment problems."

The American Workforce: A Success Story with a Price. According to Dept. of Labor statistics, the US workforce, the most productive workers in the world, have been able to generate an average of 3 per cent annual productivity increases over the last 50 years.

Remarkably enough, this annual increase has been consistent over that period of time, with the exception of a halving of annual productivity gains in the 1970s and 1980s. It is the primary reason why the American workforce remains the most productive in the world. But the progressively greater efficiency American workers have produced over several generations comes with a price tag, and the number on that tag is rapidly increasing.

The history of this amazing record of increase in US worker productivity throughout the last half of the 20th century parallels America's emergence as the preeminent economic and military power on the planet. During the first half of the 20th century, the United States labor force was transformed from a largely rural, agrarian labor force into a predominantly urban industrial worker pool. The single most significant impetus to that transformation was the Second World War.

During and after World War II, there were three major factors which combined to rapidly propel our nation to the status of global economic giant. The first was the rapid growth and transformation of the industrial infrastructure into the free world's supplier of arms and ammunition for the war effort. This infrastructure also propelled many US corporations into the global spotlight as major players on the world's economic stage. The subsequent success of companies such as IBM, Boeing, Lockheed, and countless others had their origins in those companies' contributions to the successful war effort.

The second factor was the mass relocation of millions of Americans as they enlisted for the war effort and were sent across the country for military training and, subsequently, all over the world. The lyrics of an old song from the early 20th Century captured the practical effect of this relocation: "*How ya gonna keep 'em down on the farm, after they've seen Paree?*" Indeed, the end of the war coincided with the accelerated urbanization of American society as millions of returning GIs and their families, seeking the bright lights and economic opportunity that the newly massive urban industrial base offered, rejected a return to rural life and rapidly filled up our nation's cities.

This migration was accelerated by the third factor, the large scale availability of educational opportunity through the GI Bill. Tens of thousands of American military veterans took full advantage of this program, in the process creating a much more highly educated workforce that could take full advantage of the emerging new technologies which populated the industrial landscape of that era. The benefits of these programs endure to this day: as a military veteran, I earned a professional qualification in the Boeing 737 jet airliner with the assistance of the GI Bill, joining thousands of my fellow veterans in improving my professional skills and employment prospects in the process.

The durability of the effect of these three factors is amply demonstrated today, with the US recognized as the major player in the world economy. A primary reason why we continue to enjoy this advantage is the rise in the influence of major corporations. Building on their large scale emergence in the post-WWII era, the reach of these companies into virtually every segment of American society has given rise to the label 'Corporate America.' The worker productivity statistics cited earlier could not have been achieved had it not been for the organizational structure which major corporations have been able to create and apply effectively for the collective advancement of every sector of our economy. Well run corporations offer their employees the ability to obtain job security and stability, career advancement, and a slice of the 'American Dream' for themselves and their families.

As a result, at the dawn of the 21st century, the United States stands astride the globe as the preeminent economic, military, technological and cultural superpower. Everywhere you go on this planet, you can find overwhelming evidence of the truth of this statement. No matter what country you may visit on the face of the earth, you will find large numbers of people who, for varying reasons, want to live like Americans, dress like Americans, eat and drink like Americans, and own American goods. Part of the military and cultural backlash we are dealing with in the Muslim world is due to the sheer pervasiveness of American culture. How many times have we seen film on TV of people from all over the planet wearing Levis, drinking Coke, smoking Marlboros, or eating at McDonald's? It is a primary reason why so many people seek legal immigrant status here.

While I was serving as an airline pilot, I encountered a prototypical example of an American success story, much like many of these immigrants seek to emulate. I was sitting at a hotel bar on an airline layover, having dinner with my first officer, when an attractive young woman sat down beside me. We struck up a conversation, and her moving tale transfixed me and my first officer. It was one of emigration from the Middle East with her family to escape religious persecution, arrival on the US West Coast with virtually nothing, and being raised to truly believe she could be or do anything she wanted in America. She told of how she started with a small company as a receptionist, and rose over a 20 year period to become one of its top company officers. I was deeply moved by both the fierce conviction of this woman and the empowering nature of her story.

It is due to her efforts, as well as the efforts of the many millions more who work in Corporate America, that we enjoy the many advantages and standard of living we do today. For example, walk into any upscale hotel in a large city, and sit down at the bar. You will generally see well appointed furniture, one or more state of the art TVs, a high quality music system, a menu that features food literally from around the world, a bar stocked with beverages of similar international variety, and a wait staff that efficiently orchestrates and provides all this to its customers. Walk out into the parking lot and you will see a predominance of late model cars, owned by people from a variety of ethnic, cultural and economic backgrounds.

Further, if you walk down the street, you won't have to go far to find what has now become one of America's favorite gathering places: the brand name coffee shop. Appointed more like a combination library/café, it again offers an international menu of foods and beverages served in a pleasing setting, with computer hookups or WiFi networks to boot. The same can be said of virtually any good quality restaurant you may encounter: pleasing surroundings, a varied menu, and fast service. If Americans prize one thing above all else, it's speed. Give it to me right, but give it to me *fast*.

Walk into almost any American home, and the evidence of another advantage of living in America will literally jump out at you. Everywhere you look you will see advanced technology. Whether it is microwave ovens, flat panel TVs, high tech sound systems, personal desktop or laptop computers, or portable personal electronic organizers and cell phones, we Americans love our gadgets, and use them extensively. In the process, we have influenced the entire world to emulate us.

How did this occur? Very simply, because of still another advantage of living here: scientific excellence. Since the end of World War II, our nation has pioneered stunning advances in virtually every scientific discipline. The pharmaceutical industry has produced many lifesaving drugs. The chemical products industry has rolled out brand new materials for household use. The food industry has transformed the American market, making shopping for groceries faster and more efficient than ever before.

Our scientific establishment has made breathtaking advances in virtually every arena. We have sent men to the moon, in the process revolutionizing the materials, data processing, garment and food industries. We have peered into the vastness of space with the Hubble telescope, looking backwards in time to the birth of the Universe. We have sequenced the human genome, presaging the potential end of many deadly diseases. We have harnessed the power of the atom, offering the vision of a future where energy will be virtually limitless.

Our society has become a model of speed and efficiency, providing virtually any good or service at remarkable speed. Yes, we Americans really enjoy living in our fast paced society. We use 24/7 communication, convenience stores, credit/debit cards, and state of the art technology – and we use caffeine and energy drinks, fast food and fads, diet and recovery programs, medical professionals and HMOs, and the latest breakthroughs in pharmaceuticals to help us keep up and fix us up if our bodies break down.

As our society has become more and more automated, we have also discarded one of the most healthful habits our ancestors adhered to every day: getting up and going to sleep with the sun.

Take a look at the satellite imagery below, depicting the lighted areas of Earth at night. We have truly become a 24/7 society! That transformation has brought about a very unhealthful result: sleep deprivation.

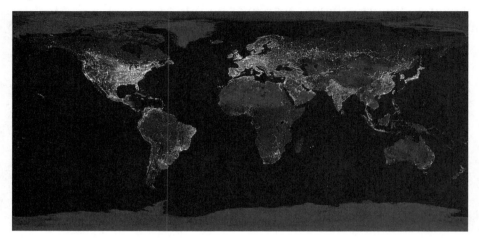

This depiction of the Earth, while admittedly beautiful, is an eloquent testament to our global civilization's determination to both provide a safe environment at night for its citizens and to attempt to increase the labor productivity of those same citizens.

Not unexpectedly, Corporate America has taken full advantage of this situation by creating a working day which now stretches literally around the clock. As we have extended the length of the effective working day, in some cases reversing day and night for many of the American workforce, we have simultaneously imposed an ever greater stress load on those same workers. The harder our society tries to become more 'productive,' the more people we expose to these conditions.

As Shakespeare famously said, "*Aye, there's the rub.*" Although we have all of these advantages as a result of our collective efforts, the unintended consequence is that they come at a price for all of us. That price? *Chronic stress*.

Government Spending and Stress: A Nation Teetering On the Brink, Fiscally and Physically. The United States government has obviously taken a significant interest in stress in that the Occupational Safety and Health Administration has declared stress a hazard of the workplace. They estimate that an astounding 43 per cent of all adults suffer adverse health effects from stress, and it is getting worse. Yet we see little or no resource allocation for dealing with chronic stress in our federal budget.

That begs the question: why is chronic stress so detrimentally impacting our government's fiscal situation? The answer lies in understanding the complex interrelationship between chronic stress, our health care system, and what portion of that system the government (meaning, us taxpayers) has chosen to address with our tax dollars.

One of our nation's preeminent stress research and reporting organizations, the American Psychological Association (APA), has helped put this connection into proper perspective. Their research has disclosed that "*extended reactions to stress can alter the body's immune system in ways that are associated with. . . conditions such as frailty, functional decline, cardiovascular disease, osteoporosis, inflammatory arthritis, Type II diabetes, and certain cancers.*"

Likewise, the National Institutes of Mental Health (NIMH) published a 2009 study that correlated chronic stress to a similar host of physical and mental ailments. And a laboratory study that looked at the effect of adrenal hormones on the size and growth rate of cancer tumor cells found a direct correlation between the presence of adrenal hormones and tumor growth.

So how does that connect with government spending? Two of the three largest items in our federal budget are those associated with retirement and health care programs: Medicare and Medicaid (the other, of course, being Social Security). It is on these two programs which we will focus our attention, because they are creating the most onerous long-term fiscal burden, characterized by virtually uncontrolled cost growth and no meaningful constraints.

Shortly after the 2008 national elections, my colleague and friend Radhia Gleis (a fellow THFC executive committee member) and I submitted a policy paper on health care reform to the newly elected Obama administration. Much of the research we did focused on this vexing problem. With thanks to Radhia for her assistance, I will share some of our discoveries here.

To begin with, the 2008 government estimate of projected annual US health care spending increases over the next decade is over 6 per cent, with some advanced health care for seniors projected to rise by as much as 70 per cent over the same period. Due in large part to the Great Recession, annual health care spending increases were below that level in both 2009 and 2010. This change has been attributed to a combination of deferred spending by consumers, who don't want to contend with potentially expensive health care bills in shrinking household budgets, and the loss of insurance by the unemployed. However, these lower rates of increase are expected to be more than made up for by an upward spike in health care spending once the economy recovers. As of this writing, the government has not released health care spending figures for 2011. In any event, by 2016, the US government estimates that health care spending in the United States is projected to reach just over $4.1 trillion and comprise 19.6 per cent of GDP. That means that in 2016 almost 20 cents of every dollar earned in this country will be spent on health care.

To put that into personal perspective, try this little exercise. If you have a five dollar bill in your wallet, take it out and lay it on the table in front of you. Think for a moment about what those five dollars could buy for you today: perhaps a specialty coffee at the local coffee shop; maybe a fast food meal; a large bottle of spring water; or even a magazine off the newsstand.

Now imagine what would happen if you only had four fifths of the purchasing power of that five dollar bill. How many of those items would you have to give up because of the decrease in purchasing power due to the increase in your health care costs?

A major portion of those costs are borne by the federal government, and directly funded by your and my tax dollars. The magnitude and direction of increase of those costs have already caused grave concern at the highest levels. For example, the US Government Accountability Office (GAO) has concluded that:

"Over the next few decades, the nation's fiscal outlook will be shaped largely by demographics and health care costs. As the baby boom generation retires, federal spending on retirement and health programs such as Social Security, Medicare, and Medicaid will grow dramatically. A range of other federal fiscal commitments, some explicit and some representing implicit public expectations, also bind the nation's fiscal future. Absent policy change, a growing imbalance between expected federal spending and tax revenues will mean escalating and ultimately unsustainable federal deficits and debt."

The GAO goes on to state that:

"Current fiscal policy is unsustainable over the long term. Absent reform of federal retirement and health programs for the elderly--including Social Security, Medicare, and Medicaid--federal budgetary flexibility will become increasingly constrained. Assuming no changes to projected benefits or revenues, spending on these entitlements will drive increasingly large, persistent, and ultimately unsustainable federal deficits and debt as the baby boom generation retires."

Effectiveness of the Current System – How are We Really Doing?
Based on the above, I think we can authoritatively conclude that
we are spending huge amounts of money (actually, too much!) on
health care in this country. Further, a growing body of research
suggests that many, if not most, of the illnesses being treated have
their root cause in chronic, unmitigated stress. But what return on
our investment are we actually getting for those expenditures?

There have been many measures used over the last century in the US
to assess the effectiveness of our health care system in addressing
the most pressing challenges facing the American people. Such
health care 'scorecards,' however, frequently employ a complex and
sometimes confusing and conflicting array of parameters to depict
this information.

In contrast, the single most widely accepted metric, at both the
national and international levels, to demonstrate meaningful change
in any nation's state of health has been the annual reporting of the
leading causes of death. In the US, this reporting began over a
century ago when the government began to gather statistics on the
various causes of US citizen deaths. As the century progressed, and
more comprehensive and sophisticated data gathering techniques
were employed, it became possible for us to draw comparisons over
time, and note the changes that have occurred.

So what conclusions can we draw from that data? According to
government statistics and supporting private studies:

*"In 2004, the 10 leading causes of death were (in rank order)
Diseases of heart; Malignant neoplasms; Cerebrovascular diseases;
Chronic lower respiratory diseases; Accidents (unintentional
injuries); Diabetes mellitus; Alzheimer's disease; Influenza and
pneumonia; Nephritis, nephrotic syndrome and nephrosis; and
Septicemia."*

Many studies have concluded that eight out of the preceding ten could
be substantially prevented through diet and lifestyle intervention.
The table on the next page depicts these causes chronologically:

Figure 1. Top Ten Leading Causes of Death in the United States, 1900 and 1950 thru 2004

Rank	1900	1950	1960	1970	1980	1990	2004
1	Pneumonia (all forms) and influenza	Diseases of heart	Diseases of heart	Diseases of heart	Diseases of heart	Diseases of heart	Diseases of heart
2	Tuberculosis (all forms)	Malignant neoplasms	Malignant neoplasms	Malignant neoplasms	Malignant neoplasms	Malignant neoplasms	Malignant neoplasms
3	Diarrhea, enteritis, and ulceration of the intestines	Vascular lesions affecting central nervous system	Vascular lesions affecting central nervous system	Cerebro-vascular diseases	Cerebro-vascular diseases	Cerebro-vascular diseases	Cerebro-vascular diseases
4	Diseases of the heart	Accidents	Accidents	Accidents	Accidents and adverse effects	Accidents and adverse effects	Chronic lower respiratory diseases
5	Intracranial lesions of vascular origin	Certain diseases of early infancy	Certain diseases of early infancy	Influenza and pneumonia	Chronic obstructive pulmonary diseases and allied conditions	Chronic obstructive pulmonary diseases and allied conditions	Accidents (unintentional injuries)
6	Nephritis (all forms)	Influenza and pneumonia except pneumonia of newborn	Influenza and pneumonia, except pneumonia of newborn	Certain causes of mortality in early infancy	Pneumonia and influenza	Pneumonia and influenza	*Diabetes mellitu*
7	All accidents	Tuberculosis	General arteriosclerosis	*Diabetes mellitu*	*Diabetes mellitu*	*Diabetes mellitu*	Alzheimer's disease
8	Cancer and other malignant tumors	General arteriosclerosis	*Diabetes mellitus*	Arteriosclerosis	Chronic liver disease and cirrhosis	Suicide	Influenza and pneumonia
9	Senility	Chronic and unspecified nephritis and other renal sclerosis	Congenital malformations	Cirrhosis of liver	Atherosclerosis	Chronic liver disease and cirrhosis	Nephritis, nephrotic syndrome and nephrosis
10	Diptheria	*Diabetes mellitus*	Cirrhosis of liver	Bronchitis, emphysema, and asthma	Suicide	HIV infection	Septicemia

*Figure 1. Heron, M. PhD, National Vital Statistics Reports, Volume 56, Number 5, Deaths: Leading Causes for 2004, 11/20/2007

These data, and much more like them, confront our nation and its leaders with an unpleasant reality: we no longer have a health care system in this country, but a disease management system, increasingly driven by the financial interests of the medical/ pharmaceutical/insurance complex and processed food industry.

I have used the term 'medical/pharmaceutical/insurance complex' as an intentional historical parallel. If you are a member of the Baby Boom generation, you may remember President Dwight D. Eisenhower's famous farewell speech on January 17, 1961. In that address, Eisenhower cautioned the nation that "*In the councils of government, we must guard against the acquisition of unwarranted influence, whether sought or unsought, by the military/industrial complex. The potential for the disastrous rise of misplaced power exists and will persist.*"

I strongly believe that we face a similar challenge today from the combination of interests of the medical profession, the prescription drug industry, and the insurance industry. Their combined influence, and their collective relationship with our government, is creating just such a situation as Eisenhower warned us about regarding the military/industrial complex over 50 years ago. Absent change, in both this relationship and the associated fiscal resource allocations it creates, the consensus among government and independent health care experts is that the size and estimated fiscal demands of the Baby Boomer population cohort will overwhelm the ability of our current health care and financial systems to meet the needs of our citizens.

The changes over time displayed in the list of the leading causes of US deaths lead to some remarkable conclusions. While we have been successful in combating communicable diseases over the last century, it is clear that we have been singularly unsuccessful in effectively combating the rapid rise, persistence and proliferation of diet and lifestyle-related diseases as the leading causes of death over the same period.

And the situation is only worsening. Please note the rapid rise in the prevalence of deaths due to diabetes mellitus (also known as adult onset diabetes, or Type II diabetes), highlighted in the chart in bold print. Virtually nonexistent before the turn of the 20th century, this illness has rapidly risen in prevalence during the last half of the 20th century. It is the fastest growing illness in the nation, and the statistics bear this out.

Among Americans age 20 and older, 142.0 million are overweight or obese. 23.6 million people—7.8 per cent of the population— have diabetes. The total direct and indirect annual cost of diabetes management efforts in the US is $174 billion. Nearly 87 per cent of adults 40 years and older are either at risk for Type II diabetes or heart disease (61.1 per cent) or have been diagnosed with one of these diseases (25.8 per cent). This presages a veritable explosion in the numbers of citizens diagnosed with diabetes in the future.

Though the medical community trumpets reductions in the numbers of deaths from each cause as evidence of progress, the durability of diet- and lifestyle-related illnesses at the top of the list, and the rapid ascent of others which were not significantly present a century ago (e.g., diabetes) minimize the validity of those assertions. The fact remains that most of the leading causes of death in the US are diet and lifestyle related. That has been the case for a long time.

Compare this list to the one cited by the APA, and the results of Holman's and Silver's post-9/11 follow up study on increases in stress-related illness. Do you see any connection? The US government does.

In *Prevention Makes Common Cents*, published by the Department of Health and Human Services, they state:

"Increasingly, there is clear evidence that the major chronic conditions that account for so much of the morbidity and mortality in the United States, and the enormous direct and indirect costs associated with them, in large part are preventable - and that to a considerable degree they stem from, and are exacerbated by, individual behaviors ... As Americans see healthcare expenditures continue to increase, it is important to focus on strategies that reduce the prevalence and cost of preventable disease."

There is no end in sight to these cost increases, which gobble up progressively greater portions of our national wealth. A big part of that increase is what we pay for pharmaceutical drugs: the top ten US pharmaceutical companies (also collectively known as 'Big Pharma') earned more in 2002 than the other 490 Fortune 500 companies combined. Largely because of these escalating costs, the Congressional Research Service labels such large scale health care spending as the single greatest threat to our nation's economic well being.

The consequences of ignoring this burgeoning threat to our physical and economic well being are now readily apparent. In addition to the dire GAO fiscal projections referenced earlier, a raft of studies has surfaced which reinforce the GAO's estimates. For example, a recent RAND Corporation study predicts that advanced health care for seniors, soon to be the largest US population cohort, will rise in cost by over 70 per cent by 2030. The study estimates that the cost of treating diet- and lifestyle-related diseases by that time will consume over three quarters of the Medicare budget. Also, the cost of drugs for cancer treatment was projected to rise by 80 per cent worldwide by 2011. Clearly, a new direction in American health care is needed to avoid this impending fiscal and health disaster.

So how does all this correlate to the prevalence of chronic stress? Let's connect the dots. The government already recognizes that chronic stress is hazardous to our collective fiscal and physical health. Credible authorities also recognize that stress is the root cause of many of the top killers in the nation and, despite the commitment of a gargantuan level of resources to treating these illnesses, we are making no significant progress in dealing effectively with them. At the same time, our government has made no substantive commitment of resources to directly address this pandemic of chronic stress.

Do the math: unless we start making smarter choices, from both a personal and governmental standpoint, *we'll never catch up.*

Stress and Corporate America: A Hidden and Growing Cost. According to a recent annual Attitudes in the American Workplace Gallup Poll, 80 per cent of American workers say they need help managing stress. Whether their employers choose to acknowledge it or not, this situation directly impacts the bottom lines of the over 11,700 publicly traded US corporations, the health of their over 102 million employees, and that of the over 5 million incorporated self-employed.

As mentioned earlier, in their book *The Stress Solution*, Miller and Smith estimate that 75 per cent to 90 per cent of visits to family physicians are for complaints/illnesses whose root cause is stress. Likewise, as Melissa Chessher demonstrated, between 7 and 9 out of 10 times a corporate employee visits the hospital, it's because of a problem due to chronic stress. This is the price we pay for progress, a price we only now are beginning to accurately quantify.

The APA, in a 2005 survey, discovered that more than 1/3 of Americans say they have had an illness that was primarily caused by stress. With the US population now sitting at over 312 million, one out of three Americans equates to over 104 million people experiencing a stress-caused illness. The APA's 2007 survey disclosed that three-quarters (77 per cent) experienced physical symptoms during the last month as a result of stress. This includes fatigue (51 per cent); headache (44 per cent); upset stomach (34 per cent); muscle tension (30 per cent); change in appetite (23 per cent); teeth grinding (17 per cent); change in sex drive (15 per cent); and feeling dizzy (13 per cent), among others.

Nearly as many (73 per cent) experienced psychological symptoms in the last month including irritability or anger (50 per cent); feeling nervous (45 per cent); lack of energy (45 per cent); and feeling as though you could cry (36 per cent). Half (48 per cent) of adults lay awake at night during the last month because of stress and on average they report losing 21 hours of sleep per month.

What is the apparent cause of this stress? The 2010 APA survey cited:

"Money (76 per cent), work (70 per cent) and the economy (65 per cent) remain the most oft-cited sources of stress for Americans. Job stability is on the rise as a source of stress; nearly half (49 per cent) of adults reported that job stability was a source of stress in 2010 (compared to 44 per cent in 2009). At the same time, fewer Americans are satisfied with the ways their employer helps them balance work and non-work demands (36 per cent compared to 42 per cent in 2009)."

The APA 2007 survey identified work related stress as the primary cause for three quarters of the respondents. The level of stress is such that half of employees surveyed (52 per cent) report that they have considered or made a decision about their career such as looking for a new job, declining a promotion or leaving a job based on workplace stress. The leading sources of stress that contribute to these decisions are low salaries (44 per cent); heavy work load

(41 per cent); lack of opportunities for advancement (40 per cent); uncertain job expectations (40 per cent); and long hours (39 per cent).

Corporate America Reacts ... But How Smartly? Many competent, prudent business managers and executives are already aware of the significance of the data presented above. The question is what have they done, or are planning to do about them. Typically, cutting costs means cutting the single biggest business expense: payroll. And that means cutting jobs.

While any astute business manager or executive recognizes that many factors impact the decision to cut jobs as a means of decreasing costs, increasingly the reason is the cost of health care. When the cost of labor in this country is examined more closely, approximately 30 per cent consists of benefits, and the bulk of that is health care costs. According to figures from the Bureau of Labor Statistics, benefits costs have increased 4.5 per cent to 7.2 per cent on an annual basis from 2004 through 2007. The major component of these increases is health care costs.

Driven primarily by these financial imperatives, our nation's corporations have, over a period of many years, sought to control health care costs in large part by increasing the productivity of their employees. In other words, by having fewer people do the same amount of work, they believe they can help better control their annual health care expenditures.

Unfortunately, despite Corporate America's and their employees' best efforts, they have been unable to generate more than an average 3 per cent annual productivity increase from the labor force, while health care costs continue to increase by over 6 per cent annually. Recent studies indicate that if this rate of increase continues, within the next five years health care will surpass payroll as a company's biggest expense. While the relationship between productivity and health care increases is not exactly linear, the point is very clear: health care costs are continuing to increase at over twice the rate of workforce productivity. The practical result is that no matter how productive a corporation's workforce becomes, they continue to fall short on an annual basis of being able to cover their own health care costs. The equally important result is an ever shrinking, chronically stressed workforce in progressively worse health and an ever growing health care bill for Corporate America.

The statistics cited above are part of an ominous trend, one which has placed Corporate America into a vicious spiral of an ever shrinking workforce and ever increasing health care costs. The diagram below helps describe this phenomenon more clearly.

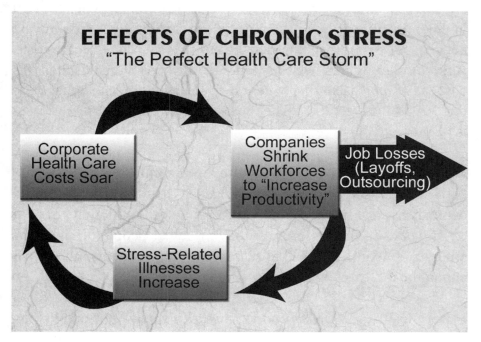

Corporate America has clearly recognized this problem, and expressed its concern as far back as 1993. A study done in response to President Clinton's proposed overhaul of the nation's health care system, largely sponsored by companies that do not provide health insurance for their employees, contended that requiring employer-paid health coverage would eliminate 3.1 million jobs. Another study, sponsored by the National Federation of Independent Businesses, stated that the plan would put 12.7 million jobs at risk and lead to one million layoffs.

More recently, a USA Today article highlighted General Motors' concern about the rapidly spiraling health care costs for its US workers. In contrast to Canada, whose national health care system subsidizes all but $120 of the benefits cost applied to each vehicle manufactured there, health care costs applied to US-made GM vehicles averaged $1,500 per car.

Health care became such a contentious issue that it contributed to the strikes at all of the Big Three automakers in 2007. Ultimately, however, the solution became a combination of job cuts and employee sharing of health care costs, a huge concession for the labor unions.

As the economy continues to globalize, the cost of American health care continues to exert a drag on our economic growth, and contributes in a major way to the loss of jobs in all sectors. For example, in 2005 Toyota decided to place a new assembly plant in Canada instead of the US. A major factor leading to this decision was the company's determination that Canada's national health system would effectively subsidize Toyota's health care costs. This factor overrode the incentives offered by the US for the company to locate here. This is but one example of a major employer bypassing the US in part to avoid increasingly onerous health care costs.

Health care costs also contribute to another, increasingly visible phenomenon: outsourcing of jobs, especially overseas. A 2003 analysis by Goldman-Sachs estimated employers shifted between 300,000 and 500,000 jobs over the past three years to such countries as India and China. The report goes on to suggest that, based on these estimates, the number of jobs sent offshore will increase to several hundred thousand annually in coming years. A 2004 study by Deloitte reported that the world's 100 largest financial-services companies anticipated the transfer of two million jobs offshore over the next five years in efforts to reduce their costs significantly. Many of the major Internet service providers have followed suit, transferring their IT and customer service functions to nations such as India, where the combination of an increasingly educated workforce, lower wages and (once again!) lower health care costs make the cost of labor much more affordable than in the US.

What are the mechanics of these decisions? As we have seen previously, a primary driver in the increase in health care costs is the stress level experienced by employees. Once corporations see their health care spending continue to rise (in large part due to stress related illnesses), they attempt to control health care costs by, among other things, reducing the numbers of workers they employ. They accomplish this by a combination of layoffs and, in many cases, outsourcing to either independent stateside contractors or overseas employees. In both of these cases the corporations do not have to pay for the health care coverage, achieving an apparent savings. The smaller workforce left behind, however, typically must now contend with an increased workload and a corresponding increased level of stress. This situation, combined with the systemic annual increases in health care costs cited earlier, sets the cycle in motion again. As corporate managers see their costs continue to rise they engage in another round of job consolidations and outsourcing, inflicting an even greater stress load on the still smaller workforce.

The evidence of this regrettable situation is apparent daily in the business pages of virtually every major newspaper, and on all the business programs of the major cable TV stations. How many times have we seen major corporations announcing job cuts or consolidations? How many times have we seen announcements of jobs being shipped overseas, or health care benefits being cut during labor contract negotiations? The inescapable fact is that we, as a nation, can no longer afford our own health care system.

The Great Recession: Making the Situation Even Worse. All of the business statistics cited previously as contributing to the level of chronic stress in America have been greatly exacerbated by the so-called Great Recession. With stubbornly high unemployment, record home foreclosures, concessionary labor contracts in both business and government, and the associated social dislocation (such as divorces and substance abuse) that results from these circumstances, we are looking at a rapidly rising and persistent level of chronic stress in this country that has never before been experienced.

The challenges presented by this situation have been recognized at the highest levels of the financial services community. Laura Choi, a research associate in the community development department of the Federal Reserve Bank of San Francisco, sounded a warning in a recent issue of Investment Review:

"Everywhere you look, the symptoms of the current recession are clear: homes lost to foreclosure, job losses across almost every sector of the economy, dwindling retirement portfolios, and frozen credit markets. But the recession has also led to a number of other symptoms that haven't been getting enough attention: headaches, backaches, ulcers, increased blood pressure, depression and anxiety, just to name a few. Extended periods of stress can take their toll on physical, mental, and emotional health, compounding the difficulties that many low- and moderate-income communities face during troubled economic times. As we think about ways to strengthen health and community development finance at the institutional level, we need to remember the impact that financial instability can have on health outcomes at the individual level."

Ms. Choi goes on to cite the findings of Paul J. Lavrakas and his team of researchers at Ohio State University. They developed the 'Debt Stress Index' to gauge the effect of worry about financial debt on health and well-being. That index reached a record high in July 2009, and has only slowly decreased since then.

Let's be very clear about the consequences of this situation. Because of our nation's inability to control health care costs, we are gradually eroding the ability of the US business community to provide meaningful employment to our citizenry. Said another way, our health care system's inability to control its costs, and Corporate America's response to that problem, are major causes of the outsourcing and outright job losses being experienced in Corporate America today. The American worker is literally being priced out of the international labor market. In turn, these factors contribute significantly to the level of chronic stress being experienced by the continually shrinking American workforce.

The worst part is that, unless something changes dramatically, *we will likely never reverse these trends.*

So here we are at the beginning of the second decade of the 21st century, literally teetering on the brink of health care and fiscal implosion, yet we still seem to be casting about for solutions. But how do we address this difficult challenge? Can we even put a meaningful dent in it? I believe we can. The way forward involves a combination of clear recognition of where we are today, how we got there, and what we need to learn and do to change things for the better. Turn the page to start the next step of our journey together.

CHAPTER 3

THE STRESS FACTORY:
A DAY AT THE OFFICE

"A human being is part of the whole that we call the universe, a part limited in time and space. He experiences himself, his thoughts and feelings, as something separated from the rest – a kind of optical illusion of his consciousness. This illusion is prison for us, restricting us to our personal desires and to affection for only the few people nearest us. Our task must be to free ourselves from this prison by widening the circle of compassion to embrace all living beings and all of nature."

— Albert Einstein

We've seen in the previous chapter how the pervasive nature of chronic stress in our society has negatively impacted our societal structures, our government, and the operation of our business community. But what about its effect on the average citizen? A key part of increasing our understanding of this aspect of the problem requires us to define who exactly we are talking about.

As mentioned earlier, there are currently over 102 million Americans employed in what we collectively call 'Corporate America.' That's due to the fact that the American economy has transformed itself over the last several decades from primarily a producer of goods to a producer of services. Correspondingly, the profile of the typical American worker has also morphed, from the factory hard hat employee to the cell phone-, Black Berry- and laptop-equipped office worker in a business suit.

Each of the many American working environments has its own set of overt or hidden stressors, and there certainly are many which have an impact on the overall state of American health. However, the overriding presence of the office worker in the American workforce, and their collective impact on the magnitude and characteristics of the resulting societal stress load mandate that we focus primarily on them.

To the uninformed observer, the typical corporate worker's environment, and the primary influences on that environment, would appear somewhat benign. However, a closer examination tells a much different and very disturbing story. A myriad of unhealthful influences combine to exert a huge, continuing and unalleviated stress load on the American workforce, in both the white collar and blue collar segments.

As a matter of course, most of us look at the situations we encounter in a typical work day and react with "*So what? That's life!*" This is because we tend to examine each of these situations, and most others that occur in our lives, as individually and linearly occurring events, having at most an indirect or sequential connection with one another. Many of us will readily agree we do things we know aren't good for us, such as eating doughnuts or staying up late at night, but we justify them as being the exception, not the rule, and that "*this one little thing won't really hurt us*" in the larger scheme of things. This reasoning conceals from us the resulting impact on our health, and the fact that these factors don't act linearly, but cumulatively, in concert and often unabatedly. Usually, there is no attempt by the American corporate employee, or their bosses, to "*connect the dots.*"

If we were able to accurately assess the impact of stress on our lives, to take each of these individual scenarios and situations that we think we can handle so easily, and multiply the tiny, incremental effects of each of them as they occur, thousands of times over our lifetime, we would come up with dramatically different answers than we do now. That's because it is the cumulative effect of each of these scenarios and situations that creates chronic stress and its devastating effects. To gain a better appreciation of what this combination of stressors does to the human body, let's closely examine what an office worker encounters during a typical day on the job in what you will soon see can be accurately called "*America's Corporate Stress Factory.*"

Starting Our Day: A Morning Ritual That Adds to Our Stress. As a society, we have been conditioned to perform certain daily routines which are considered simply a part of 'getting ready for the day.' The application of grooming products like deodorant or hair spray, each laden with synthetic chemicals of one kind or another, is an example of this cultural conditioning.

We are all familiar with the more sensational examples of the effects of chemical exposure that have been splashed across the mainstream media over the years. Stories about the effects of coal dust on West Virginia coal miners ('black lung' disease), asbestos poisoning on construction workers (mesothelioma) and, more recently, the sensational stories about the fatal side effects of certain prescription drugs have conditioned the public consciousness to accept that chemical exposure in large doses is toxic to the human body.

What has been missing until recently, though, is an examination of the effect of small, persistent, incremental chemical exposure over a lengthy period of time. We are only now beginning to understand that this type of exposure can be equally harmful. For example, the recent findings that many people suffering from Alzheimer's disease have very high concentrations of aluminum in their bodies and brains has turned the scientific community's investigative focus to whether long-term, chronic exposure to aluminum sources such as aluminum-based anti-perspirants or cookware is the culprit.

While the state of this scientific research, and others like it, is not yet settled, some alarming trends are already apparent. For example, it has been estimated that, as a species, mankind has been exposed to more new chemical influences in the last fifty years than in its entire history prior to that. Further, it may surprise you to know that as little as a trillionth of a gram of any substance is enough to start a low level hormonal reaction in the body. Is it any surprise, therefore, that chemical exposure, regardless of the individual dose, is a major stressor in our society? When we take into account the cumulative nature of this exposure, not only from examples like that above, but also from activities like the regular refueling our car, the ever growing stress load we are imposing on ourselves becomes increasingly apparent.

The Workday Begins: Wading Through Traffic. Let's look at another influence on the American corporate worker, one to which anyone living in or near a large city can relate: traffic jams. While all city dwellers have come to expect slowdowns in urban traffic flow at various times of the day, it's when the traffic slows to a crawl, usually at a time when we feel we can least afford it, that the sub optimization aspect of our society rears its annoying little head again, much to our self-perceived detriment.

The engineers who design the incredibly complex and (usually) efficient highway system of a city do so under very tight fiscal, time and space constraints. They use a number of different parameters to accomplish this demanding task, not the least of which is an estimate of the anticipated traffic flow on that highway. In a society with unlimited resources, we could expect the engineers to tailor their design to handle *any* anticipated traffic demand. However, each municipality expects its highway system to occupy the least amount of space practical, for both economic and aesthetic reasons, and to cost the minimum amount necessary. Therefore, building the most capable system is usually out of the question. So the engineers have to make tradeoffs, usually by designing a system which can handle the *average* traffic flow throughout a given day. However, anyone who has sat in their car through a big city rush hour knows that the traffic flow at that time is anything but average.

Now let's throw in a new wrinkle: one of our fellow commuters has had to drop off her child at day care and is late getting to work. So, she drives down the traffic choked highway *just a little bit faster*, her heart racing. As she looks at her watch to ensure that she's still on time, someone else abruptly moves into her lane and brakes hard in front of her. The result: a classic fender bender that completely shuts down that major highway and brings traffic flow to a standstill. As a result, many, many more commuters are now placed in the situation where *they* are late for whatever appointments they must meet, and each of them reacts with varying degrees of anger, frustration, and venting. As a result, their bodies kick into a stress response.

Corporate Office Buildings: An Overlooked Stressor. After fighting our way through the morning traffic, we arrive at our corporate offices. In most cities, these buildings are typically multistory or high rise, steel framed buildings with central climate control. Therein lie two of Corporate America's most widely experienced but least recognized stressors.

In Chapter 1, we discussed the effect of the metal cage of a high rise office building on our body's electromagnetic field. One-time or infrequent exposure to this environment is obviously not harmful. But repeated exposure to this environment consistently distorts the body's vibrational field at the DNA level. It therefore cannot help but distort critical cell functions and processes, and therefore the operation of the body's systems which are comprised of those cells.

Another likely contributory factor to this problem is the central climate control system that typically conditions the air of these buildings. Although the technology of central air conditioning has improved dramatically over the last several decades, a design feature it has been unable to avoid is that it is still essentially a closed system. This certainly offers the advantage of shielding the occupants from unhealthy outside influences. However, because of the huge size and complexity of the system's plumbing, it also ensures that anything already trapped in the system will likely remain there.

While the filtration system can efficiently eliminate dust particles or small particulates like smoke, it does little or nothing to affect the ability of microscopic particles like bacteria, fungi or viruses to survive, or even thrive. And since the size and complexity of the system's plumbing makes it virtually impossible to keep the entire system completely clean, there is always a risk, some would say a certainty, that these illness- and stress-causing 'critters' are wandering around these systems, offering an opportunity for corporate employees to increase their likelihood of illness and therefore their stress load.

The Office Break Room: Stressors Lying In Wait. Once we arrive at our office, most of us begin our workday by heading for the break room and grabbing either a cup of coffee or a soda, and perhaps a morning snack or pastry to help us start our day. The common elements of most of the beverages are two of Corporate America's most widely used beverage ingredients: caffeine and artificial sweeteners. What most people aren't aware of is that these 'crutches' actually *increase* the stress load on the body, in the process contributing greatly to the problem of chronic stress in our society. Of these means which our society uses to cope with stress, by far the most prevalent are caffeinated beverages.

The coffee and soft drink industries, the world's two largest producers of caffeine-laden products, have invested billions of dollars in the continued production and consumption of their products. In fact, coffee is today the second most widely cultivated crop in the world! Likewise, the diet product industry, a heavy user of caffeine, invests huge sums of money in the manufacture and promotion of its products. Small wonder, then, that we hear so little about the detrimental effects of caffeine from these industries or the studies sponsored by them. You'll recall we addressed the absolutely critical issue of the monetization of American science, which has a profound and direct impact on the quality and accuracy of the information we receive about health, in Chapter 1.

Given all of the above, how can we tell if caffeine is really good for us? An examination of the body's reactions to caffeine tells the true story. We should emphasize at the outset that caffeine is a drug. A member of the methylxanthine family, caffeine attaches to the same cell receptor sites as heroin and cocaine. The supposed 'energy boost' one feels after ingesting caffeine is actually the tension felt by the body as it deals with caffeine. The reaction of the body to caffeine can be summed up as: Caffeine = Stress.

In his landmark book *Caffeine Blues* (listed in the Resources section), Stephen Cherniski states that caffeine, a direct adrenal gland stimulant, is consumed on a daily basis by over 200 *million* Americans. Since the body's primary means of managing stress is the adrenal glands, it should therefore come as no surprise that, according to stress expert Datis Kharrazian, DC, "*Adrenal disorders are probably the most common functional disorders found today.*" In his best-selling book, *Adrenal Fatigue*, James Wilson, DC, ND, adds that "*it's estimated that up to 80 per cent of American adults suffer some level of adrenal fatigue at some time during their life, it remains one of the most under diagnosed illnesses in the US.*" Chronic caffeine use/abuse is a major contributing factor to the prevalence of these functional disorders. Combined with our previous discussion in Chapter 1, all the above leaves no doubt that regular caffeine use is a source of chronic stress.

Whether they use caffeinated beverages or not, many other employees of Corporate America use various types of 'diet' beverages in an attempt to avoid the calories contained in beverages sweetened with processed sugar. The common ingredients in most of these sweeteners are either aspartame or Splenda®.

Commonly known as NutraSweet®, Equal® or Spoonful®, aspartame is one of the world's most widely used artificial sweeteners. Originally discovered in the late 1960s, it is currently used in over 5,000 food products and available in over 90 countries. But what effect does it have on the body's stress response?

Like my examination of caffeine, I discussed the in depth effects of artificial sweeteners in a Chapter 1. As if that wasn't enough, consider this: continual aspartame use has been convincingly linked to a host of serious diseases, and over 90 adverse physical reactions, most having to do with interruption of normal brain chemistry. In fact, 80 per cent of the registered consumer complaints to the FDA on food or additives in 1997 concerned aspartame, and that trend continues today. It is obvious, therefore, that aspartame contributes greatly to the chronic stress load on our bodies.

An increasing number of people have become aware of these detrimental effects, and so elect to consume only products sweetened with the newer artificial sweetener, Splenda®. After all, the thinking goes, the manufacturers advertise Splenda® as being "*made from real sugar.*" True enough, but it's what they *don't* tell you about the ingredients that is even more important. Part of Splenda's® manufacturing process involves the introduction of chlorine into the chemical mix. If you know anything at all about chlorine, you know that, in either its liquid or gaseous form, it is very antagonistic to the proper functioning of the thyroid gland, the organ of the body that helps regulate our metabolism.

Once we select our beverage of choice in the break room, most of us turn to the vending machines to select a food product to go along with our beverage. While some corporations are beginning to offer healthy alternatives, e.g., fruit bowls, in their employee break rooms, the vast majority of food choices are high calorie, processed food products. The common denominator here is usually high carbs and/or the previously mentioned caffeine. By that, I *do* mean chocolate! As mentioned in Chapter 1, the combination of caffeine and theobromine in a 3 ounce chocolate bar makes it the caffeine equivalent of a large mug of coffee. Additionally, the high carb content of most vending machine foods plays havoc with your blood sugar. Look at it this way: how many times have you experienced the 'sugar high,' followed by the 'sugar crash?' Again recall our discussion of this in Chapter 1. But don't take my word for it: does not your own bodily reaction in this situation convince you that this is stressful?

Our Work Station: An Ergonomic Stressor. Having chosen our food and drink, we sit down at our desk, and the presence of another significant source of stress becomes apparent. Many of us are already familiar with the condition known as 'carpal tunnel syndrome,' a decidedly 21st century injury brought about by (you guessed it!) chronic stress to the hands and wrists. The business world has responded to the prevalence of this condition by offering preventives such as ergonomically correct computer keyboards, but the ergonomic stress of the work station goes much further than that.

As I will detail in later chapters, a primary means of stress alleviation is regular aerobic exercise. In contrast, even a perfunctory examination of the corporate office work station clearly shows that it is (inadvertently) designed to promote immobility. At the same time, the uneven availability of ergonomically correct office furnishings, from desks to sideboards to chairs, adds to the likelihood that a person's unique musculoskeletal structure will interface imperfectly with their office environment. The result? Back, hip, neck and shoulder pain, all stressors of varying degrees.

How does this affect productivity at work? A 2004 study published in the American Journal of Psychiatry showed that back pain was a leading cause of lost productivity (i.e., absences and shortened work days) in the work place, among a population of sedentary office workers. Obviously, the work station can be convincingly included as a major source of stress.

The Electromagnetic Office Environment: An Invisible Stressor.
As we look around our work station, another stressor rears it head. Whereas our 'metal cage' office building exerts a relatively passive but significant physiological effect, the collection of electronic equipment we surround ourselves with creates a decidedly active combination of electromagnetic fields which interact with us down to the cells deepest within our bodies.

Make no mistake: our 21st century civilization could not offer the combination of goods and services, and do so with such remarkable speed, without the assistance of these marvels in electronic engineering. Tracing their development to the miniaturized transistors perfected for use in the nation's Apollo space program, our cell phones, desktop and laptop computers, personal digital assistants, as well as the servers and networks that support them, are indispensable elements of the infrastructure that services Corporate America.

But, like everything else, those advantages come at a price, one that is only now becoming apparent. For years, a few courageous scientists and researchers, led by the pioneer George Carlo, PhD, have warned about the hazards of unshielded cell phones. Hired as a consultant to the cell phone industry in the early 90s, Dr. Carlo was supposed to produce research that proved unrestricted, unshielded cell phone use was completely safe.

To his surprise, and the consternation of the industry, the results of that research proved exactly the opposite. Dr. Carlo attempted to alert industry heads to this hazard; for example, in a letter to one company CEO, he pointed out "*an emerging and serious problem concerning wireless phones.*" The research conclusively showed, via digital thermography, that as little as a one time exposure of 15 minutes to cell phone radiation, via a cell phone held close to the ear, created dangerous changes in cellular temperature deep within the brain, setting the stage for, in the worst scenario, brain cancer.

Unfortunately, due to the financial stakes involved, his words fell on deaf ears, and the industry attempted to cover up and discredit his research. Since that time, however, a growing chorus of voices has joined Dr. Carlo's, raising awareness in the general public that unrestricted use of unshielded cell phones poses a major health risk.

One of the most significant voices is Vini Gautam Khurana PhD, an Australian researcher who recently completed a 14 month study involving review of over 100 sources in the most current medical and scientific literature, in addition to press reports and Internet content. Dr. Khurana presents alarming evidence concerning a cell phone's effect on the body, adding further that "*its effects on the body, particularly its electrical organ, the brain, are compounded by numerous other simultaneous long-term exposures including continuous waves from radio and TV transmitter towers, cordless phone base stations, power lines, and wireless/WiFi computing devices.*" This accurately describes the typical office environment, replete with all the devices mentioned above, making it clear that this segment of our workplace is a major added stressor.

Hand in hand with this stressor is the continuing and ever-accelerating advance of the complexity and sophistication of our electronic devices. Desktop/laptop computers, hand-held digital assistants and cell phones do, indeed, allow our professional lives to be more productive. However, that same complexity and sophistication requires us to perform more mental work to ensure we are using these devices most efficiently. As I point out in more detail in the section below, these almost constant 'mental gymnastics' have been proven to be another major source of stress.

Other Corporate Workplace Influences: The Stress Piles On. Let's look at a few more examples of stressors in the office environment. A virtual prerequisite in Corporate America, unless you happen to own your own company, is the interface between you and your employer. With few exceptions, most Americans approach their jobs with the attitude that, for whatever reason, they want to do as good a job as they can. The motivation may simply be the need of a living wage, but frequently also includes the prospect of higher wages, a potential promotion, personal recognition, or simply being able to hold onto the job, period. It's really immaterial which of these it is: in the minds of most people, doing the job well is important. However, how they do the job can be a source of contention with their employer, and therefore of stress for themselves.

In the current corporate environment, the twin priorities are quality *and* quantity. It's not enough anymore to simply do the best job we can; we've got to do it quickly and correctly the first time so that we can move on to the next task, do that quickly and correctly the first time, etc. This pressure to continually outperform yourself is ever-increasing, and never-ending. The added stress is that, with the company's emphasis on continually increasing productivity and holding down cost growth, if we aren't able to adequately produce, we're gone after the next performance appraisal. In some companies, that occurs as frequently as every 90 days. Because our lifestyle, and that of our family, is directly tied to our ability to earn a living wage, the stress becomes more complex, i.e., we not only worry about holding onto our job, but also about whether we can manage financially.

Because the corporation's primary emphasis (some would say its *sole* emphasis) is to continually increase employee productivity, some interesting 'rules of the game' have evolved in the workplace over the last several decades. For example, it was once universally recognized that an employee with personal challenges at home sometimes needed a reasonable amount of time away from the workplace to deal with those challenges, so they could quickly return to their workplace and focus on being more productive.

Although many companies today still allow for these circumstances, that is by no means the universal standard. In stark contrast, many corporations expect their employees to remain productive *in spite of* any personal challenges at home. While the employee may be encouraged, and even expected, to bring extra work home to continually increase productivity, they are definitely *discouraged* from taking any time away from the workplace to deal with personal challenges. In the extreme, this has frequently resulted in employee termination. When this is a prominently visible factor in the workplace, it can only add, incrementally but significantly, to the stress load.

Unfortunately, as a result the average corporate employee is caught in a trap of the body's own making. As the workload continues to increase, the ability of the employee to use his/her higher mental functions such as judgment, creativity and decision making, becomes progressively less influential (more about that important subject later!). The body's stress response kicks in, and all of a sudden, it's a fight for survival; it's just as if we were being chased through the forest by a saber tooth cat, only this time the predator is our in-basket.

Faced with these challenges, the workforce in Corporate America resorts to many techniques and gimmicks to maintain the pace required today. One of the most prevalent is multitasking, the management of several tasks simultaneously.

On the surface, this appears to be a viable strategy. Armed with the latest in technology, the corporate employee can certainly keep track of several tasks and functions at once. Indeed, the ability to multitask is a prized talent in Corporate America. But does multitasking truly allow us to operate more efficiently? The research reveals some surprises.

A revealing summary of the effects of non-stop multitasking is contained in Walter Kirn's November 2007 article *The Autumn of the Multitaskers* in the magazine *The Atlantic*:

"*Multitasking messes with the brain in several ways. At the most basic level, the mental balancing act it requires – the constant switching and pivoting – energizes regions of the brain that specialize in visual processing and physical coordination and simultaneously appear to shortchange some higher areas related to memory and learning. We concentrate on the act of concentration at the expense of whatever it is that we're supposed to be concentrating on.*"

In other words, as long as our activities involve *doing*, we can cope with the situation. However, when we must shift to thinking, our performance degrades if we're multitasking. As we will see in a later chapter, this is a primary manifestation of the body's stress response.

Kirn's conclusions are supported by another recent article, posted on the web site of the American Psychological Association. Titled *Is Multitasking More Efficient? Shifting Mental Gears Costs Time, Especially When Shifting to Less Familiar Tasks*, it validates and supports Kirn's statement. Apparently, our brains use different sets of rules, which activate different parts of our brains, when performing different tasks. It is this shifting between rules within our brains that takes time, the result being that we *think* we are being more efficient, but in actuality are not. The unfortunate reality, though, is that we definitely do add to our stress load.

Another way corporate employees increase their productivity, as mentioned earlier, is taking work home with them. Since our family obligations are also important, and take up a given amount of time at home, the only time these employees can find to accomplish this extra work is at night, when we would normally be asleep. I alluded to sleep deprivation as a cause of stress in the previous chapter, but that discussion told only part of the story.

We now have the capability to turn on the television or computer at any time of the day or night and access literally thousands of entertainment options, or to go out on the street and enter clubs, shops and restaurants until the wee hours of the morning. Not unexpectedly, Corporate America has taken full advantage of this situation by creating a working day which now stretches literally around the clock.

As we have extended the length of the effective working day, in some cases reversing day and night for many of the American workforce, we have simultaneously imposed an ever greater stress load on those same workers. What has been the impact? A 1996 study, jointly conducted by NASA and a major cargo-carrying airline, disclosed that the average life expectancy of cargo plane pilots who flew night schedules for most of their careers was decreased by an average of *five years* in comparison to their day-flying coworkers.

Every night shift worker, no matter what he or she does, is subject to these same debilitating factors. The only difference is a matter of degree. The harder our society tries to become more 'productive,' the more people we expose to these conditions. For the people who are continually exposed to these conditions, they are a continuing source of stress.

Unfortunately, the effects of our 24/7 society go way beyond a simple shortening of life spans. The health care industry has watched with varying degrees of alarm over the last several decades as our young girls have begun menstruation at earlier and earlier ages. There are a couple of factors at work here: one is the prevalence of xenoestrogens (chemicals which react in our bodies like the hormone estrogen) in our society; they have an accelerating effect on sexual development. But equally influential is the gradual speeding up of our biological clocks by the change in the ambient light levels of our civilization. Some studies now contend that, due in large part to around-the-clock light exposure, the daily circadian rhythm has decreased to as little as 20 hours; the implications for all of us are sobering. Assuming this data is accurate, it means that for every ten calendar days we live, we actually age twelve days. For every month we live, we age 36 days. For every year we live, we age a year and one fifth. For every decade we live, we age 12 years!

Sleep deprivation causes a whole host of additional problems which have been addressed in many well written books: decreased productivity; weight gain due to increased consumption of sugar laden 'energy' foods; increased usage of caffeine containing foods and beverages; increased susceptibility to accidents, are among the major factors. Taken together, our stress load climbs even higher.

Another way corporate employees attempt to increase their productivity is to work non-stop in the office, without taking any breaks. Just keep the coffee cups filled and they can work all day, right? Well, not really. We saw earlier how detrimental chronic caffeine abuse can be, but that's only half the story. It is the demand that we maintain our attention to the tasks at hand for extended periods of time, sometimes for hours on end, which equally stresses us.

One of the benefits I experienced as a military veteran was exposure to the US Air Force's superb training system. As a B-52 pilot, I was trained to operate some of the most complex and lethal machinery on the planet, tasks far more demanding than those required of most office workers. It comes as a surprise to most people, however, that the Air Force typically structures this complex training in fifty minute blocks, with ten minute breaks in between. Why? Because the Air Force long ago figured out that a person's attention span in a learning environment, and therefore their productive activity, was limited to about fifty minutes without a break. Any longer, and the body's stress response kicks in to help maintain attention, depriving the brain of full access to its higher mental processes. Why, then, do we see thousands of workplaces where breaks are severely limited, or non-existent? Count this as a major source of workplace stress.

Corporate America and the Standard American Diet (It Really Is S.A.D.!) We've made it through the morning, and now it's time for lunch. Many inveterate multitaskers will use this opportunity to attempt to be more 'productive,' eating at their desk while continuing to work. We've addressed this productivity illusion earlier. The focus here, though, is on what we put into our bodies.

Whether we use this opportunity to overstuff ourselves, thinking (erroneously) that we need the extra food to 'keep going' through the day, or we elect to 'keep it cheap,' with an eye on better managing our financial situation, a frequent common element is our selection of fast food.

A headline above an online news article said it all not long ago: *The US Is Eating Itself To Death.* The article went on to describe the soaring rates of obesity, the prevalence of 'super size' portions in fast food restaurants, and the effect this all has on our nation's collective health. But does it contribute to stress? Absolutely! Let's look at just a few aspects of our nation's dietary habits to gain a better perspective.

Because we are such a clock-oriented society, we have fallen into the trap of believing that the less time we spend on any given activity, the more efficient we have become. This belief (another of Deepak Chopra's 'hypnoses') has given rise to the huge number and variety of fast food restaurants. You are undoubtedly already aware of the best-selling book *Fast Food Nation*, which is listed in the Resources section, but it is important to understand how this aspect of our dietary habits contributes to the epidemic of chronic stress in our society.

When you look at the S.A.D., number one on the culprit list is certainly fast food. The primary stressors in these food sources are the types of foods (usually high calorie, high fat), the chemical soup that usually accompanies them in the form of preservatives, additives and pesticides, and the predominance of partially hydrogenated fats (also known as trans fats). These foods all contribute to stress, but the trans fats are definitely the worst. Their effect on the heart aside, and as mentioned in Chapter 1, they literally rob our body of the raw material we need to deal effectively with stress.

Hand in hand with fast food go high carbohydrate foods; sometimes they are one and the same! These foods act as 'rocket fuel for the body,' causing our blood sugar and insulin to skyrocket. We may feel really good for a while, because they are processed in the body so fast. But then, just like a rocket that doesn't reach orbit, our blood sugar will come down really fast, too! Unfortunately, high carbs have a very detrimental impact on the body's ability to handle stress, as well as greatly overstressing the pancreas.

A new wrinkle in the products that now line our grocery shelves is so-called Irradiated Food. The reason the food manufacturers came up with this idea was to allow a food to remain on the shelf longer without spoiling. Well, they can certainly do that. However, the process of irradiation does a couple of very unhealthful things to these products, and I'm not talking about adding radiation! First, it literally destroys the nutritional value of the food; what we eat has about the same value as cardboard. Second, it also destroys the enzymes that would otherwise exist in the food. These enzymes are what cause the food to spoil, but they are also critically important to our ability to use the food in our body when we eat it. Enzymes are the 'chemical engineers' that allow the food to break down in our digestive system so our body can use its nutrients. Foods that contain no enzymes require our body to use its own enzyme reserves to digest it. Since most people are enzyme deficient anyway, by eating irradiated food we're literally running our body out of the very thing it needs most to use food properly.

We all enjoy attractive looking food on our plate. But do we really know how it got that way? Much of the produce that is organically grown does not look particularly attractive when compared to the 'normal' produce in the grocery store. That's because the 'normal' food has, in many cases, been treated with chemicals and dyes to enhance its shelf appearance. Combine this with the fertilizers and pesticides used to grow and protect it, and we're in effect ingesting a chemical soup which plays havoc with our cellular metabolism and the functioning of our organ systems.

All of these factors come together with a vengeance in the food selections offered in most public settings. Grocery stores, restaurants, convenience stores all share the blame, but airports take the cake. When's the last time you saw real, healthful food in an airport? To the extent we routinely expose ourselves to this type of nutrition, we continue to add to our stress load, sometimes daily, for years on end.

Our Stressful Relationships, In the Office and Out. We all derive at least some stress in our lives from the fact that we humans are social beings. By our very nature, we seek companionship of and association with other humans. For the majority of us, our closest relationships are with members of our own biological family. These relationships hold the potential to offer both the most nurturing behaviors in our lives *and* the most destructive. When the latter overwhelms the former, we experience stress, and that stress can easily spill over into the workplace.

As an example, I offer my own family's experience with my late brother. From a very early age, Sean was an obviously gifted athlete. His skills ranged from tremendous foot speed, to a rifle of a throwing arm, to a kicking foot that rivaled many pro football punters and place kickers of the time. However, as we found out much later in his life, Sean was afflicted with a learning disability; he was dyslexic. Back in the 1950s and 1960s, when the three of us siblings were moving through our primary and secondary education, there was precious little awareness, much less commitment of resources, devoted to children with Sean's challenge.

Most families, my own included, dealt with children like Sean as 'problem' students lacking motivation. Since both my sister and I were honor students, unflattering comparisons were drawn between Sean and us by both our parents and our teachers. By the time his grade school years were over, Sean's labeling, by teachers, family and himself, as 'slow' and 'dumb' was deeply ingrained. The stress this inflicted on him was enormous, contributing in a major way to both his promising but failed athletic career and his eventual descent into the nightmare world of addiction to drugs, alcohol and tobacco. Although he experienced mixed success with recovery from drugs and alcohol, it was his chronic, lifelong tobacco addiction that finally claimed him. He died of lung cancer in May 2006 at age 53.

Much of Sean's addictive tendencies were reinforced by the modeling behavior offered primarily by our father. A lifelong smoker himself, Dad smoked around us from a very early age (like Sean, his smoking was a major contributing factor to his death from recurrent prostate cancer in 1996). I credit his offering me a puff on his cigar during our 1956 summer vacation as being the primary motivation for me to never use tobacco again; it tasted *awful!* Sean, however, picked up on the literal interpretation of Dad's modeling (*"Do as I do"*) and began smoking at age eight. When children received mixed, confusing modeling messages from their caregivers (*"Do as I say, not as I do!"*), it creates stress.

Additionally, we are all familiar with the phenomenon of someone close to us 'pushing our buttons,' i.e., greatly annoying us by the way they interact with us. This type of behavior by our family members can range from teasing to disparaging remarks to, in the extreme, abusive behavior toward us. If this occurs on a frequent or recurrent basis, it adds significantly to the stress load.

As we continue to develop physically, mentally and emotionally throughout our childhood and teen years, the modeling behavior of our peers begins to occupy a preeminent place in our value system. This is especially so during our teenage years, when the natural process of differentiating ourselves from our parents, as well as from their values and expectations, exerts a powerful influence. With the overlay in our current society of the enormous pressure for teens to engage in high-risk behaviors (i.e., illicit drug use, promiscuous sex, etc.), the stakes have become extremely high. To the extent that there is a conflict between what our parents expect and what our peers demand, our chronic stress load is added to even more.

All of this forms the background for each employee who enters the corporate workforce today. An underlying, foundational concept of family systems theory contends that, when you interact with any fellow employee in a business setting, you are interacting not only with him/her at that moment, but with the sum of the experiences and influences of that person's lifetime up until that moment.

A related dynamic also occurs when a person enters the work force. Because of the structure of the corporate workplace and the method of interaction between and among coworkers and supervisors, there are many elements in common with both the family and peer group settings. Therefore, depending upon the workplace scenario, an employee can face a combination of family and peer interactions, both positive and negative, when dealing with his/her coworkers. Overlay this with the inevitable influence of office politics and you have one more source of stress to deal with.

An additional, unique input occurs in the office setting from the employee's supervisor. Many times, this can be a very positive experience, especially if the manager is cognizant of the importance of a motivational leadership style and has the latitude to employ those skills to the benefit of the company and its employees. However, if the company culture is excessively focused on results, and management views its employees as simply vehicles to achieve those results, the working climate can be positively miserable.

During the course of my 20 year military career, I had the occasion to work for both types of leaders. I found it interesting that the bosses who achieved the most allowed their subordinates the latitude to assume responsibility and accountability. Everybody won.

Conversely, the leaders (and I use the term loosely) who focused solely on results and frequently used the expedient negative motivational techniques of fear, sarcasm and ridicule achieved some results, but none which equaled the true leaders. There is a long-standing joke in the military about the effectiveness of this so-called expedient leadership style. To the extent that this style truly prevails in a corporate workplace, the workers are constantly exposed to stress, and are truly less productive as a result.

Corporate Travel: A Major Source of Stress. As our economy has continued to globalize, Corporate America has responded by increasing the mobility of progressively greater segments of the American workforce. Just take a look at the passenger loads at most major airports, especially on the heaviest travel days of Friday and Sunday. Travel has become an indispensable element of business today.

It is equally important, therefore, that I share some of my personal combination of experience as both an airline pilot and traditional naturopath. With some business travelers spending almost as much time 'on the road' as they do at home, they approach the environmental stress load that airline flight crewmembers (pilots and flight attendants) experience as a matter of course throughout their careers. In fact, airline crewmembers and, by extension, frequent business travelers are routinely exposed to one of the most toxic environments on the planet. That may seem a bit counterintuitive, given the almost sterile working environment passengers observe. Let's take a closer look.

First, airline crewmembers and frequent travelers are constantly exposed to changes in their circadian rhythm. Circadian rhythm is the cycle of day-night, waking-sleeping, that is supposed to be governed primarily by the rising and setting of the sun. Most people's daily routines provide a relatively stable circadian rhythm upon which their bodies rely for a whole host of functions. Not so for airline crewmembers and their best customers. Every time they go to work on a schedule earlier or later than 'normal,' or cross one or more time zones, the 'internal clock' of their biological rhythm gets a little messed up. When the number of time zones crossed exceeds three, they experience the phenomenon known as jet lag.

During my 16 year airline career, I both commuted to work every week and crossed multiple time zones virtually every trip. I can tell you from both personal and professional experience that this has a long-term, detrimental impact on one's state of health.

Many thousands of years ago, the Chinese discovered that each organ system performs specific functions at specific times of the day via this internal biological clock. For example, according to the Chinese clock, the large intestine, or colon, experiences its greatest activity from 5am to 7am; the bladder, from 3PM to 5PM: and the gall bladder, from 11PM to 1AM. When we move the body to a different time zone and have no way to adjust our body's internal clock, confusion results. That is why international travelers, and the crews who serve them, experience the 'not right' feeling associated with crossing multiple time zones; their biological clocks are not in sync with the time associated with their position on the earth.

Most people would view this situation as a mere inconvenience; the research says otherwise. Every time our circadian rhythm is disrupted, it is a stressor. Since stress is cumulative, the effect can be lasting and significant. Although every person is affected differently, some sobering conclusions have already been drawn.

As mentioned earlier, a study conducted by the pilots' union at a major cargo carrying airline discovered that the difference in life expectancy between those who flew a day schedule most of their careers versus those who flew nights was five years. The night flyers were on the short end of the stick because of the constant readjusting their body clocks had to undergo (i.e., normal daytime schedule at home, 'backside of the clock' nighttime schedule at work).

Second, *every* crewmember or passenger, regardless of what time of day they fly, is exposed to high altitude radiation. Flying at altitudes between five and eight miles above the earth deprives the human body of the vast majority of the protection that earth's atmosphere provides at sea level. For example, at 18,000 feet, half the atmospheric protection is below us. But at 41,000 feet, over 90 per cent of the protection is below us. Those international travelers and crewmembers who routinely fly the international routes over the poles are at even greater risk because they fly through a portion of the earth's atmosphere where the tropopause, the last layer of atmospheric protection, is thinner than elsewhere.

However, *every* passenger or crewmember who flies in an aircraft repeatedly at high altitude is continually exposed to some degree. How much? Research conducted by Dr. Jesse Stoff, M.D., a prominent immunologist, disclosed that the average radiation dose on a cross country flight equaled that of a *chest X-ray!* Multiply that by several dozen or more times per year, and we begin to get the picture. A lifetime career in the airline industry exposes crewmembers to *thousands* of times the normal lifetime radiation dose of an earthbound human, or even the frequent traveler.

Third, everyone on an airliner, passengers and crew alike, is exposed to some degree to the noise generated by both the aircraft engines and the high speed airflow around the aircraft as it travels through the sky. There is a large body of well-accepted scientific knowledge that convincingly documents the hearing loss and accompanying fatigue caused by repeated exposure to this type of noise. This helps explain the growing popularity of the use of noise canceling headsets on airplane flights by both passengers and pilots. Obviously, repeated exposure to this type of noise falls into the category of chronic stress.

Fourth, the pilots flying those aircraft, as well as those passengers and crew sitting toward the front of the plane, are constantly exposed to electromagnetic (EMF) radiation from the aircraft avionics and cockpit instrumentation. In the Boeing 737, the aircraft in which I have logged most of my flying hours, the pilots sit right above the avionics compartment; there is no shielding. Every flight, we get a dose of EMF from in front, behind, above and below us. Combine that with the high altitude radiation mentioned previously, and is it any wonder that airline pilots are among the highest risk groups for brain cancer and leukemia?

Fifth, every airliner is equipped with a combination re-circulating and ram air, air conditioning system. While this minimizes the likelihood of toxic fumes intruding from outside the aircraft, it also ensures that almost everything that is already inside the aircraft stays there. Despite the fact that the system is equipped with a capable filtration system, it cannot filter out the microscopic viruses and bacteria that passengers bring on with them.

This creates problems any time of the year, but it is especially bothersome during cold and flu season. So, every flight, everyone on board is exposed to the totality of the airborne bacterial and viral load the passengers have boarded the aircraft with. In many ways, it's like flying in a 100 foot long, aluminum Petri dish. The Federal Aviation Administration (FAA) *has* recently commissioned a study group to examine the problem of air quality in airline cabins, but a comprehensive solution is many years away.

Sixth, that same air conditioning system also filters out virtually all of the humidity in the re-circulated air, forcing passengers and crewmembers alike to fight a constant battle against dehydration. The in-flight humidity in the cabin and cockpit is on the order of 5 per cent, much like you would experience in the high desert of the western US. That means that on every flight, every crewmember and passenger is losing a significant amount of water simply by evaporation through the skin. While exact data on water loss is not currently available, the magnitude is on the order of many ounces during a long distance flight.

Finally, while on the ground, the aircraft is usually cleaned with some mix of chemical cleaning solutions, and with the doors open, passengers and crew are exposed to the fumes from the jet fuel-powered auxiliary power unit that provides ground air conditioning and electrical power. A single exposure to this environment would not normally be harmful. Again, it is the cumulative load of each individual exposure, multiplied by hundreds of times every year that subjects people to significant, comprehensive toxic stress.

Loneliness in the Workplace: An Unexpected Source of Stress. On the surface, one would think that, with all of the devices at our disposal which increase connectivity, we would feel an increased sense of fulfillment and connectedness in our business and personal relationships. Unfortunately, the reality is otherwise. The more time we spend interacting with machines, the less we interact with real people. This lack of personal interaction has definite, negative physiological consequences. The September 2007 issue of the online journal *Genome Biology* detailed a study that showed loneliness depresses cell sensitivity to key adrenal hormones and actually makes you less able to respond positively to stress. This research was so groundbreaking that *Discover* magazine declared it one of the top 100 science stories of 2007.

Home After a Hard Day: Relaxing, or Adding More Stress? To our collective credit, most of us Americans recognize that chronic stress has a detrimental impact on our lives. And building on our forebears' heritage of self-reliance, we have tried mightily to correct the problem ourselves. Unfortunately, the 'solutions' many of us have attempted to use have only made the problem worse. Let's look at some of the more prevalent ones.

One of the Usual Suspects: Alcohol. A widely accepted means our society uses to relax and 'de-stress' at the end of a workday is through consumption of alcoholic beverages. Most of us are well familiar with the societal challenges we face in dealing with chronic alcohol abuse. There are many authoritative books on this subject and I will not attempt to detail their conclusions here. A common recommendation is that moderate alcohol use (one to two drinks per day, depending upon the type of alcohol consumed) is healthful. But one area that these experts ignore is the effect of even moderate alcohol consumption on the body's stress response.

In its most elemental form, alcohol is a sugar, the most highly refined form of sugar available in any food or beverage. Because of its fermentation, alcohol's initial effect on the body is depressive, i.e., people feel more relaxed. However, introduction of processed/ refined sugar of any type into the body causes the adrenals to release hormones called glucocorticoids (otherwise known as cortisol) to aid the body in the processing and absorption of the alcohol. This acts as a stimulus for the adrenal glands. Over time, regular consumption of alcoholic beverages can result in 'rebound effect' later on at night, causing the person to awaken and disturbing the natural sleep cycle. Obviously, for this and many other reasons, alcohol also adds to the chronic stress load we must deal with.

Lighting Up to Relax: Need I Say More? While we are all grateful that tobacco use in this country has decreased to less than one quarter of the adult population, that still means that many tens of millions of Americans continue to use this incredibly harmful substance. For over forty years, the US government has preached the dangers of smoking and its correlation to lung and other types of cancer. I've already shared the story of my brother's and father's demise due to smoking; to that I can add my grandmother (stomach cancer) and aunt (chronic leukemia). All of them were regular smokers whose illnesses were either directly caused by or contributed to in a major way by their tobacco habit. Their collective experience, and that of many people we all know, point to the additional hazards of smoking.

First, nicotine is addictive; despite the efforts of Big Tobacco to minimize the portrayal of this effect, in many ways it acts as a drug. Second, it is *extremely toxic*. Cigarette smoke deposits significant quantities of cadmium, a toxic heavy metal, throughout the body, but especially in the lung tissue. A major contributor to the eventual development of lung cancer, emphysema and related diseases is the poisoning of lung tissue that occurs at the hands of this extremely dangerous toxin. Third, most smokers, because of their diminished lung capacity, are unable or minimally able to take advantage of regular exercise, a primary means of normalizing the stress response. For these reasons and a host of others too numerous to mention, nicotine is a major source of stress.

Sitting Down at the Dinner Table . . . or Not. A major change in American society that has evolved over the last couple of decades is the virtual disappearance of the family dinner. Where once this was the sole opportunity for meaningful family communication and reinforcement of family cohesion, the gradual and inexorable filling up of each family member's activity calendar, children included, has by default created a situation where each fends for themselves. This forces family heads to provide meals that are quick and easy, and not necessarily nutritious. Despite the fact we have already fed (and I use the word loosely!) ourselves with fast food for the morning and lunchtime meals, we again create a scenario where our bodies are offered food that may be filling, but is not giving us what we truly need to operate these incredibly complex organisms efficiently. It is the difference between what we eat, and what our bodies really need, that creates one more significant source of stress.

Household Chores: "Push A Button And It Goes" - How A Leisure Lifestyle Creates Stress. It is very likely that, after dinner, we also have to deal with a myriad of household chores that require our time, effort and attention. As a society, we have become almost addicted to the labor saving devices that make these chores easier and quicker to accomplish. We are truly a gadget loving nation, taking great enjoyment in "*push the button and it goes.*"

The next time you sit down in an airline cabin for a flight, take a moment to look at the catalog in the seat back pocket in front of you. It is chock full of descriptions of devices that are the fulfillment of "*push a button and it goes.*" Paging through the publication reveals floor washing robotic vacuum cleaners, remote control golf balls (!), self-pumping garden sprayers, and a host of other devices. While the exact task we are avoiding varies with each device, the common element is "*you don't have to exert yourself.*"

Each of these devices, and many others like them in households throughout America, do indeed perform valuable functions. Collectively, though, they have helped to create a mindset in our population characterized by a woman who visited our booth at a health expo. Her question was typical of the mindset of so many people in this society today: "*how can I lose weight and not have to exercise?*" This mindset is a crucial contributor to the problems we have with chronic stress.

Intertwined with this problem is the fact that, as we have become increasingly dependent on these devices, we have become less and less movement oriented. During each airline trip I have flown, I have seen innumerable elderly (and quite a few not so elderly!) people sitting in wheel chairs in our airports. While the specifics of each person's health challenges differ, the common element with many if not most of them is that they didn't get up and get moving early enough in their lives to avoid being immobile now. The lack of movement now inflicts a whole host of other health problems on them. Combined with the draconian measures (such as drugs and surgery) they must now endure to stave off even worse ill health and function at all, we can say with absolute certainty that these people are dealing with enormous chronic stress.

Mass Media: Stress Brought Right Into Your Living Room.
When we finally finish the after-dinner chores, we slump into our favorite easy chair and turn on the news. How many times have we commented to our family, friends and coworkers that *"they always seem to report only the bad news?"*

Having grown up in a broadcast media family (my Dad was a TV broadcaster and show host for a local New York City TV station for over 40 years and, prior to their marriage, my Mom was a time buyer for NBC Radio), I was able to see this dynamic at work firsthand. The TV stations we watch are, like any other businesses in this country, in existence to make a profit. They spend an incredible amount of time and effort fine tuning their programming to meet the expectations of their target audiences, and rely on a number of different measurement tools to determine what types of programming satisfy their audiences' desires.

In the case of news reporting, whether it is TV, radio, or print, the time-tested adage that governs content is *"bad news sells."* As a result, with few exceptions we can expect to see the most violent, lurid, or scandalous items leading the reporting on a nightly news program or on the front page.

With the advent of 24 hour cable news channels, the competitors have taken this paradigm to an even more intense level. How many times have we turned on one of the 24 hour news stations, only to see words like *"News Alert,"* *"Developing Story,"* etc., all accompanied by attention getting warning tones and/or music that makes our heart race? Suddenly, it's as if we are actually there in combat in Afghanistan or Iraq, at the site of a new earthquake, hurricane or forest fire, or in front of the courthouse confronting a newly convicted corporate bandit or mass murderer. We alluded to this same phenomenon as adding to our societal stress load after the events of 9/11.

When we're finished with the news, we usually turn to our favorite nightly TV programs. A quick look at the weekly Nielsen ratings, the primary gage of TV viewership in this country, reveals a predominance of 'action,' 'suspense' or 'reality' programming. We get an 'adrenaline rush' watching programming where the outcome is in doubt, where the protagonist is in danger, and where the finale usually ends with some sort of violence or action to resolve the episode's plot. While we find this type of entertainment enjoyable, make no mistake. It activates the same systems in our bodies that being chased down a forest trail by a saber tooth tiger does.

Many younger people choose instead to immerse themselves in the dizzying array of video games available today. Again, the predominant type of these products emphasizes action or violence, in some cases very graphic violence.

The fidelity of these products, in terms of the computer generated imagery, sound effects, and general plot line, is such that they have the power to generate a very visceral response from most people using them. I have stood over my own son's shoulder on occasion, watching him play an interactive World War II combat game; even after watching for a few minutes, I felt my own body responding to the action on the screen.

The realism and intensity of these game scenarios, while entertaining, holds the potential to create a chronic response in an individual playing the game over and over again. Some of the other games on the market, especially fantasy adventure games, are even more intense. There is emerging research that shows that people who play these games repeatedly (usually young men) become more and more predisposed to violent behavior themselves.

Some of these same games have an interactive component involving multiple players on the Internet. The Worldwide Web, while offering us access to an incredible array of information, also holds the potential to contribute to the problem of chronic stress. Many Web surfers spend endless hours at their computers, sometimes late into the night, thus contributing to the previously mentioned problem of sleep deprivation. Research shows that this occurs because the light energy emitted by high fidelity computer monitors stimulates a portion of the cortex of the brain that, after about 9PM, leaves the brain in an excited state where it is very difficult to relax enough to be able to sleep. Combine this situation with already stimulating content on the computer screen, and it's small wonder that 'surfing the Web' now qualifies as a stressor.

Opening the Mail: Interacting With the Other End of Corporate America. Before we address the work we brought home from the office, we frequently engage in one of the most common American end-of-the-day rituals: opening and responding to the daily mail. It is here that the confluence of the monthly bills, the constraints on our earning power, the resultant limits on our ability to provide for ourselves and our families, and the stressful climate of our nation's financial management system come home to roost, in a very personal way. If we are already immersed in financial difficulty, or even just teetering on the brink, this can be among the most stressful activities of the day.

Frequently, opening the mail also involves a phone call to a customer service department of a corporation to solve a problem with a product or service we have purchased or utilized.

We have all had the occasion at one time or another to call the customer service number at a company whose products or services we have purchased. Because of the way the customer service function at corporations has evolved, we can expect to wait on hold for several minutes when we do this. (*"Thank you for calling XYZ Corporation's customer service center. Your call is very important to us. All our customer service representatives are busy serving other customers. Please do not hang up. Your call will be answered in the order received. We apologize for any inconvenience. The expected waiting time is approximately ten minutes."* Click. Segue to Musak.)

When we look past the superficial aspects of this situation, we can find a very interesting dynamic at work. The corporation is responding to its own set of stressors in this scenario. On the one hand, it would like to serve its customers in a timely manner so that it can preserve its reputation and continue to be profitable.

At the same time, it must respond to the demands of its shareholders to control costs and limit expenses. Since one of the most expensive items on its balance sheet is employee benefits (as mentioned in Chapter 2), it must walk a very careful line between providing acceptable customer service and controlling the costs of providing that service. Therefore, in the ultimate it must decide how much waiting time is acceptable for its customers, and then decide how many employees it needs to fulfill the goal of not exceeding that waiting time. In other words, it must decide how much of its money it must spend to limit the amount of time we spend on the phone waiting.

However, since we usually are calling about an issue or problem that has arisen with its service or product, we approach it from an entirely different viewpoint. If our time is limited, e.g., we are making the call after work and just before we must pick up the kids at soccer practice, *we expect to not wait at all.* After all, it is the company's product/service that has gone awry, so why should we now have to waste our valuable time waiting to address a problem that's the company's fault to begin with?

So we sit there, fuming and checking our watches, seeing the time we must leave to pick up the kids rapidly approaching, simply because XYZ Company won't hire any more customer service reps. *This heartless, impersonal, inconsiderate company obviously thinks their money is more important than my time!* As we continue down the track associated with that train of thought, we can feel our bodies respond to the feelings those thoughts generate. That response is stress.

Checking E-mail and Starting the Take-Home Work: Sub Optimization Comes Full Circle. Finally, we are ready tackle the twin tasks of responding to our daily e-mails and then digging into the take-home work from the office. In so doing, we confront the structure and function of a technological innovation which has become indispensable in our society: the personal computer.

As I fired mine up today to start writing this portion of the book, I was confronted with an array of messages: *"Internet Access Updates are ready to install,"* *"Welcome to Windows Update Manager,"* *"Your Anti-Virus Software Subscription Will Expire in 14 Days,"* etc. *I only wanted to check e-mail and start writing again!* Each of these programs obviously serves a valid and useful purpose on my personal computer. Without them, it would be at the mercy of a host of problems that are beyond my personal ability to solve. However, the very fact that they each were developed and written by separate organizations means that, by their very nature, they interface imperfectly with each other, with my computer hardware and, most importantly, with me. While I appreciate and enjoy the advantages each of these programs offers, their imperfect 'fit' with each other creates an ongoing intrusion into my ability to use my computers when I want, how I want. Although this is usually a relatively minor inconvenience, it is an ongoing, long-term, cumulative one, and to that extent, is a source of stress.

Chronic Stress: A Matter of Connecting the Dots. As we have seen, a close examination of the typical corporate work environment clearly demonstrates that daily, incremental chronic stress ripples through our business community at every level, created by the food choices we make, the resultant nutritional deficiencies, the lifestyles we choose, our own thought patterns, and toxic influences, all of which are byproducts of our advanced society.

Because most of us operate by extrapolating our linear thinking, we therefore come to the erroneous conclusion that if our bodies can handle each of these situations individually, we must be able to handle all of them at once and indefinitely, right? *WRONG!* Our bodies are designed to handle moderate stressors from any one or a mix of these categories for a brief time, but they are not designed to handle a group of high level stressors all at once for an extended period of time.

But in order to find out why and, even more importantly, what we can do to change our self-destructive situation, we need to understand more clearly the operation of our endocrine or glandular system. This system, and its component parts, are truly the body's energy managers, the arbiters of how our bodies' finite energy resources are used. Turn the page to continue your journey of discovery.

Part Two

How It All Works:

Creating the Stress Stack

CHAPTER 4

THE BODY'S ENERGY MANAGERS:
A LIMITED LINE OF CREDIT

"Sometimes it is more important to discover what one cannot do, than what one can."

— *Lin Yutang*

The Endocrine Co. If you are employed by one of the many entities and organizations that comprise Corporate America, you are undoubtedly familiar with the typical 'wiring diagram' organizational chart that depicts the corporate hierarchical structure. In their best-selling book, *The Starfish and the Spider*, authors Ori Brafman and Rod A. Beckstrom describe this type of hierarchical organization as a 'spider' organization, needing direction from the top in order to thrive. If the leadership of the organization (i.e., 'the head of the spider') is removed, all integrated control of the organization ceases, and chaos results.

Our body's endocrine, or glandular system operates in much the same way. It has a 'front office' of sorts that directs the functions of the other glands in the system, telling them when to turn on and off. The 'department heads,' the other glands, are each assigned tasks (the operation of one or more of the body's systems) and given resources (the body's energy stores) to accomplish those tasks.

Another feature of this system is that, just like a corporation, the allocation of those resources shifts when a crisis presents itself. How many times have you seen a corporate department receive the lion's share of available resources on an emergency basis, simply because their assigned task is the most time or mission critical? Well, the endocrine system operates just like that.

So, as we explore the body's endocrine system, we will continue to use this analogy between its operation and that of a typical corporate structure. We will, as a result, avoid the linguistically and conceptually complex scientific descriptions that usually accompany such discussions. In the process, however, it is my hope that all of you will gain a more functionally oriented comprehension of one of the most important systems of your body.

Some Basic Terminology. When someone refers to "*the endocrine system*," what exactly are they talking about? Mosby's Medical Encyclopedia describes it as follows:

"*Endocrine system*, the network of glands . . . and other structures that secrete hormones into the bloodstream. They affect the function of specific target organs. Glands of the endocrine system include the thyroid and the parathyroid, the pituitary, the pancreas, the adrenal glands, and the gonads. . . Secretions from the endocrine glands affect a number of functions in the body, [such] as metabolism and growth. Endocrine glands also affect secretions of each other and of organs."

There are a couple of important concepts that need to be addressed here, and I will continue to use the business analogy to do so. First is that every company's goal can be distilled down to its mission statement. In each case, the further distillation of the mission statement usually translates to 'inflow exceeds outflow.' In other words, the resources the company receives (i.e., its profits) exceeds the resources the company expends (i.e., the money it spends to acquire the resources it needs to produce the products or services it sells).

Second, if the company encounters difficulty in the business world, it can usually operate for a short period of time in an emergency response mode, typically in a condition where it is operating at a loss. The company's ability to do so will be completely dependent upon its operating reserves. However, if it is not able to exit this emergency response mode within a short period of time, it usually declares bankruptcy and ultimately, can go out of business. So it must use its finite input resources efficiently in order to accomplish its mission.

The body's endocrine system operates in a similar manner. The body receives a finite amount of resources (i.e., the food it uses to create energy) to operate its systems. Usually, this operation takes place in an environment of equilibrium, what the medical community calls "*homeostasis*." The endocrine system is what the body uses to manage the expenditure of this energy source.

The body does have an emergency response system, also known as the stress response, to allow it to operate for brief periods in a sort of 'overdrive.' If the response operates for only short, infrequent periods, the body is able to return to equilibrium quickly and continue to operate healthfully.

However, if the body continually uses this 'overdrive' function, it will quickly use up its energy reserves. Then, like a company whose financial reserves are exhausted, it slips into its own form of bankruptcy, what the medical community calls disease. If the conditions causing the bankruptcy are not effectively addressed, then we become the fulfillment of *chronic stress decreases the age at which we die*.

But how does this system actually work? To understand, let's use a corporate analogy that we're all familiar with: the computer local area network, or LAN.

If we work in virtually any corporate office setting, we typically each have a desktop computer or terminal of our own, hooked up to a sometimes complex network of wiring (or a wireless network, in more sophisticated settings), and a central server or servers that permits us to communicate directly with other computers, and peripheral devices such as printers. Each computer or terminal may or may not be individually turned on and off by the operator.

The 'LAN' that operates the endocrine system is indeed centrally controlled by its own 'servers,' two organs called the hypothalamus and pituitary gland. None of the other glands have a 'switching' system that is integral to each, so they have to rely on the 'front office' of the hypothalamus and pituitary to tell them when to operate.

Also , they operate like a LAN system that has specific software for each terminal, allowing certain terminals to communicate with certain other terminals, but only at specific times and under specific conditions.

Very much like the operation of a computer LAN, the endocrine system requires expenditure of the body's finite energy resources to operate properly. As long as an office LAN has electrical power available, it can operate effectively. But introduce a power failure, and all activity stops.

Likewise, the endocrine system both manages the body's energy bank, and expends some of that energy in the process. It operates like an integrated LAN, controlling the level of energy expenditure of each device (gland) hooked to the LAN so that each activity can occur at the appropriate time.

In doing so, it demonstrates the last part of Mosby's description: *"Endocrine glands also affect secretions of each other and of organs."* In other words, like an advanced LAN, the connection among all the glands in the system demonstrates that one has an effect on all.

There are a great many specific, complex biochemical interactions among the glands that allow them to interact usefully and healthfully with each other. I promise you, we have no need to delve into those complexities! At this point, the most important thing to note is that, as a system, they act in concert to manage the body's expenditure of available energy.

An Endocrine Co. 'Department' Overview. Taking the corporate analogy one step further, let's take a trip to The Endocrine Co.'s corporate web site 'home page.' We'll click on the *"About Us"* link, and learn a little more about the 'departments' that comprise this system.

The 'Front Office.' The endocrine 'front office' is actually composed of two organs, the hypothalamus, and the pituitary gland. Mosby's defines the hypothalamus as follows:

"Hypothalamus /hi'pothal'ms/, a portion of the brain, forming the floor and part of the side wall of the third ventricle. It activates, controls, and integrates part of the nervous system, the endocrine processes, and many bodily functions, [such] as temperature, sleep, and appetite."

It's important to note that the hypothalamus is a rather unique organ in the body. It functions as part of both the nervous system and the endocrine system. As we can see from the definition above, it is involved with a wide range of bodily functions. We will not go into detail describing every function here, but it is important that we spend a little time discussing the hypothalamus' function in managing the endocrine and nervous systems.

As part of the role it plays as the 'chairman of the board' in the endocrine 'front office,' the hypothalamus acts as both a sensor and an activator. By that I mean that it first senses the level of each hormone in the body and, if the level of that hormone is low, sends a signal to activate that particular gland, or the central nervous system, as the situation requires. However, the signal doesn't go directly to the gland in question.

The hypothalamus communicates its messages to both the nervous system and another organ in the brain called the pituitary gland. We'll again use Mosby's definition to continue our discussion: "*Pituitary gland*: The small gland joined to a gland (hypothalamus) at the base of the brain. It supplies many hormones that control many needed processes of the body. . . The pituitary gland is larger in a woman than in a man and becomes larger during pregnancy."

The pituitary gland has also been called the 'master gland,' because it exercises direct control over all the other glands in the endocrine system. Like the hypothalamus, the operation of the pituitary gland involves some incredibly complex biochemistry, but the important thing to remember is that the pituitary gland is the 'CEO' of the endocrine system. It directs the operation of the entire system. In the process, it also determines how the body's available energy resources will be allocated, both for what purpose and for how long.

There is also a key concept that merits explaining to understand the importance of the hypothalamus and pituitary gland. As the 'front office,' these two organs use discrete channels of communication for each endocrine gland, called the control axes. When health care professionals describe these axes, they usually include the name of all three organs in the description. Each of these control axes is associated with specific hormone secretions, and bodily functions that occur as a result of those secretions. For example, when describing the mechanism that controls the adrenal glands and the body's stress response, the term used is "*the hypothalamus-pituitary-adrenal axis*," also abbreviated HPA axis.

Meet the Department Heads. Each endocrine gland acts as the equivalent of a corporate department head. Just like a company, each department (gland) performs very specific functions that are critical to the overall effectiveness of the 'company.' We'll spend just a little bit of time on each of the other glands before we get to those dealing with our stress response. It is important to do so because it will contribute to our overall understanding of the profound nature of our body's stress response.

The 'Metabolism Department.' One of the most critical functions that the human body performs is metabolism. Once again, Mosby's offers an easy-to-understand description:

"*Metabolism* , the sum of all chemical processes that take place in the body as they relate to the movement of nutrients in the blood after digestion, resulting in growth, energy, release of wastes, and other body functions. . . Exercise, body temperature, hormone activity, and digestion can increase the rate of metabolism."

It may not seem apparent that all of that definition is important to understand but it is. Said another way, metabolism governs the body's energy production processes. These are the processes that provide us the energy source for all our body's functions and activities.

The second part of the definition highlights the interdependent relationship of metabolism and the other major body functions. This interdependence is a crucial concept that underlies the systemic nature of the body's stress response.

The body's metabolic processes are controlled by the thyroid gland:

"*Thyroid gland, thyroid*, an organ with many veins. It is at the front of the neck. It usually weighs about 30 g. It is made up of bilateral lobes connected in the middle by a narrow connection. . . The thyroid gland is slightly heavier in women than in men. It becomes bigger during pregnancy. The thyroid gland releases the hormone thyroxin directly into the blood and is part of the endocrine system of ductless glands. . . Its removal greatly lessens the oxidative processes of the body. This causes a lower metabolic rate characteristic of hypothyroidism."

As this definition implies, the thyroid is critical to normal metabolism. The key idea to keep in mind is that the thyroid gland controls the rate of the metabolic processes in the entire body. If its functions were to be eliminated or impeded by removal of the organ, disease, or a chronic stress response pattern, the body's metabolism would slow down, causing weight gain and a host of other health problems.

The 'Digestion Department.' A major contributor to the success of the 'Metabolism Department' is the system of organs which control and facilitate digestion of food, the raw material for producing the body's energy. Within the endocrine system, the primary organ that assists this process is called the pancreas: "*Pancreas* /pan'kre-s/, a fish-shaped, grayish-pink gland about 5 inches long that stretches across the back of the abdomen, behind the stomach. It releases insulin, glucagon, and some enzymes of digestion. . . insulin. . . helps control the body's use of carbohydrate. . . glucagon. . . counters the action of insulin. . . enzymes. . . help digest fats and proteins."

In combination, these three products of the pancreas help to facilitate the use of the raw material (food) needed by the body to produce energy at the cellular level. We will delve into the importance of this organ in the stress response a bit later.

An important additional concept to understand is something called "*insulin resistance.*" This condition can occur for a number of reasons, but the one we are most interested in is the presence of chronic, unabated stress. In this case, the constant demands being made by the body as it deals with stress create a situation where the cells need more and more glucose to function, but the ability of insulin to facilitate glucose transport is significantly diminished. This occurs because, over time, the constant barrage of insulin against the cells' membranes causes those membranes to actually oxidize.

A useful analogy is a drain pipe covered with a screen mesh. As long as the screen remains clear, water can flow through the pipe. But if the screen rusts (oxidizes), the water flow can be significantly diminished. That 'rusting' is what happens to a cellular membrane when insulin resistance occurs. We will explain the relationship of insulin resistance to chronic stress in the next chapter.

The 'Reproduction Department.' Another important part of the endocrine system is the reproductive system: "*Reproductive system, also called genital tract.* The male and female sex glands, nearby ducts and glands, and the outer sex organs."

These organs produce the reproductive hormones estrogen, progesterone and testosterone in varying quantities, depending upon the gender of the person. There are a couple of very important concepts we need to understand about the reproductive hormones that have to do with the stress response.

First, the reproductive hormones, like the adrenal hormones cortisol, DHEA and aldosterone, are synthesized from the same source of raw material. That source is the cholesterol manufactured by the liver, which is then transformed into the pre-hormonal substance pregnenolone. This class of hormones is called steroid-based hormones. Again, we won't go into complex biochemistry here!

Suffice it to say that there is a finite supply of this hormonal raw material, and the body's internal processes, including the stress response, use it wisely.

Second, the biochemical pathways that ultimately result in the production of both the reproductive and adrenal hormones allow for some interchangeability. This makes perfect sense when we recognize that the stress response is in fact the body's survival mechanism. The body therefore has multiple means of providing itself the hormonal raw material it needs to fuel that response.

While any reproductive hormone could conceivably be transformed by the body into an adrenal hormone, the one which is most easily used for that purpose is progesterone. As such, to use an athletic analogy, I call it the 'pinch hit' hormone, filling in on a temporary basis when there is a shortage of adrenal hormones. This idea will be important to understand when we move to the next chapter.

The 'Crisis Management' Department. This is the part of the 'company' that is literally responsible for the survival of all the remaining 'departments,' and helps us deal with chronic stress. If a company in the business world detects a threat to its existence, it mobilizes all its available resources to combat or avoid the threat. In many cases it shifts resources from other departments to the part of the organization that is responsible for meeting the threat, to ensure that it will survive in the face of the threat.

That is also the case with the 'crisis management department' of the company that is the human body. And the star players of the 'crisis management department' are two, thumb sized organs called the adrenal glands.

The word adrenal is the combination of two word roots: "ad," which is Latin for "*on top of*"; and "*renal*," which means "*concerning the kidneys.*" So the combination literally means "*on top of the kidneys.*" Mosby's defines the term as follows:

"*Adrenal gland*, the organ that sits on top of each kidney. The gland has two parts: the cortex and the medulla. The adrenal cortex secretes the hormones corticosteroids [primarily cortisol, DHEA and aldosterone; author insert added] and androgens. The adrenal medulla makes epinephrine [otherwise known as adrenaline; author insert added] and norepinephrine." Two additional facts are important to note. The hormone cortisol plays a major role in both supporting blood sugar management and combating pain and inflammation, and the hormones aldosterone and epinephrine help manage blood pressure. More about those functions later.

If you've ever been involved with a business in crisis, you know that it cannot operate indefinitely in that mode. The allocation of resources in crisis mode is radically different than it is in normal, day-to-day operations. Resources which are shifted to combat the crisis must be returned to the departments that normally use them in order for the business to continue to survive.

The 'Endocrine Co.' operates in much the same way. The stress response is, pure and simple, the body's survival mechanism. When it detects a significant threat to itself, it then prepares for either a fight to the death or a headlong flight from likely destruction by a foe it perceives as superior to itself.

The Rev. Wayne Muller, in his wonderful book, *Sabbath*, offers a stark and meaningful description of what happens when we ignore this important fact:

*"We do not feel how much energy we spend on each activity, because
we imagine we will always have more energy at our disposal. This
one little conversation, this one extra phone call, this one quick
meeting, what can it cost? But it does cost, it drains yet another
drop of our life. Then, at the end of days, weeks, months, years, we
collapse, we burn out, and cannot see where it happened. It happened
in a thousand unconscious events, tasks, and responsibilities that
seemed easy and harmless on the surface but that each, one after
the other, used a small portion of our precious life."*

Given the obvious consequences of ignoring Rev. Muller's advice,
it's therefore extremely important to understand what the normal
stress response is intended to do for our bodies. First, *it is designed
for brief, intense response*, such as 'fighting/fleeing the saber tooth'
like our ancient ancestors did. A quick burst of activity to fight or
flee the threat is what the human body is designed for.

Second, it requires *specific physical activity* to normalize the body
once the response is activated. Again, our ancestors physically,
aerobically exerted themselves to either fight or flee the threat and
normalize their body's responses. The interrelationship between
this physical activity and the ability of the body to recover cannot
be overemphasized!

Third, stress *exerts a cumulative effect on the body* if the response
is not normalized. In other words, 'a couple of weeks off' won't
suffice! As mentioned previously, Stephen Cherniski's *Caffeine
Blues* describes this phenomenon as the 'vacation illusion.' Most
people believe that a relaxing vacation of a couple of weeks' duration
is all they need to restore their bodies to normal functioning.

In truth, however, given the stress load most Americans carry today,
that two week vacation offers at most a brief and temporary respite
from the continuing growth accumulation of their personal Stress
Stack. Within a short time after returning from their vacation, they

are back on the treadmill, moving their bodies closer and closer to the catabolic threshold and their eventual descent into exhaustion and, ultimately, overt illness.

Fourth, stress exerts a *systemic effect, affecting virtually every bodily system.* We'll take a closer look at that in just a minute. It's literally like dropping a pebble in a pond. The effects ripple throughout our bodies to its deepest levels.

Fifth, the stress response *is physiologically supportive for only a short time.* Since it's designed for brief, intense bursts of activity, and to be normalized shortly thereafter, the body can only sustain itself healthily if it's exposed just briefly. As such, if the opposite, chronic response is allowed to continue, it will therefore be destructive over time.

Finally, *when the stress response is allowed to degenerate into a chronic pattern, it sets the stage for serious physiological breakdown.* Said another way, *chronic stress increases the rate at which we age, and decreases the age at which we die.* It's that simple and that powerful.

But how does our body undergo this remarkable transformation? When a person experiences stress, the brain responds by initiating about 1400 different responses including the dumping of a variety of chemicals to our bloodstream. This gives a momentary boost to do whatever needs to be done to survive.

It's also important to recognize that our body's stress response is very ancient. How ancient? Allow me to introduce you to one of our ancient ancestors; see if you can relate to her experience:

A'nath'a's Story.

Location: A forest in the northern hemisphere of Pangaea (what is now south central North America)
Time: approximately 12,000 years ago

It had been a good gathering, and A'nath'a was pleased with the large number of roots, tubers and plants in her sack. The clan would enjoy a good evening meal tonight, if the men were able to match her success in gathering with a productive hunt. Despite her relatively young age, she was acknowledged as the expert in this important area of clan life, and reveled in the recognition it brought her.

She smiled to herself as she thought of the increasing attentions of Daorth, but she was in no hurry to take a mate. She enjoyed the freedom of being able to come and go as she pleased, roaming an ever larger area around the clan's caves, exploring the varied terrain and familiarizing herself with the new and interesting plants she discovered.

More than once, she had found that these plants possessed properties which could help heal a wound, break a fever, or soothe a bruise. She knew that her skills were an integral part of the success of the clan, and felt a strong sense of obligation to continue to expand her knowledge in this area.

The forest trail along which she moved with an easy, loping trot was surrounded on either side by a riotous profusion of color, although predominated by varying shades of green. Majestic fir trees soared into the canopy above her, combining with the somewhat shorter but bushier live oaks to create a dappled net of light and shadow that seemed to keep the forest floor in perpetual motion.

At ground level, the lower slung cedar plants hid much of the surrounding terrain from view, but enough of the ground cover was visible to present a rainbow of beautiful flowers scattered like a living carpet over the forest floor. The cool morning breeze wafted the fragrances of each of the flowers across her path, making the journey home all the more pleasant.

The familiar feel of her soft, loose fitting leather tunic was comfortable in the shadiness; she knew that if she stayed away too long from the cave the rising summer heat would quickly become stifling. All the more reason not to delay her return. She shifted her long shafted wooden spear with its large flint head from her right hand to her left and continued homeward.

A'nath'a moved confidently along this familiar trail, her hide-clad feet navigating deftly over and around the few logs and rocks which crossed her path. The clan had done a good job of clearing this part of the trail; it made the return that much easier.

She looked curiously at one of the tall pine trees as she strode by; struck by lightning from a recent storm, it was literally cloven in half, one part of the large trunk having peeled away from the other like a fruit rind, embracing an adjoining tree with its boughs like a child grasping its mother. She estimated that enough of the damaged tree was intact that she could clamber up to where the two trees touched and climb the rest of the way into the undamaged tree. She would be rewarded with a panoramic view of the surrounding forest.

What a wonderful way to spend a day! In the same instant she knew the experience would have to wait; the clan was expecting her.

Rounding the next bend of the trail, she skidded suddenly to a stop, her heart pounding. No more than three handfuls of paces ahead of her, standing astride the trail, was the largest Long Tooth she had ever seen.

The cat stood crosswise at the top of a slight rise, looking directly at her. Its massive, low slung body rippled with innate muscular strength. Clear, cold, yellow eyes regarded her with increasing interest; long fangs glinted in the dappled sunlight.

A'nath'a knew immediately that, with the wind at her back, the cat already had her scent. Her every muscle tensed. Instinctively, she hefted her spear above and behind her head. Her eyes widened and her breath quickened. She had only two choices: either stand and fight, or run for safety. But where? Immediately, she envisioned the split tree, a few handfuls of paces down the trail. If only she could get there . . .

As if reading her mind, the cat lithely slid directly onto the trail facing her, its limbs smoothly and powerfully moving into a low crouch. A deep, guttural growl echoed across the forest as its massive fanged head lowered to the ground. Its nose continued to move as it absorbed her scent. A'nath'a knew without a doubt now: she was its prey.

In an instant, her decision was made: RUN! Before the cat could approach further, she wheeled rapidly around and sped back down the trail. If only she could reach that tree! She heard the deep, bellowing roar of the cat in response, and sensed that it was already in pursuit. Her blood pounding in her ears, she saw the split tree just a few paces ahead. Almost there ... ! In response she heard another roar, closer this time.

As she reached the base of the tree she stole a quick backward glance. It was nearly on her! Dropping her spear, she clambered up the damaged trunk and heard another snarl. Another glance back and she screamed; it was climbing too!

Quickly, she scrambled up the rest of the way to the branches which overlapped the adjoining tree. Reaching desperately for the nearest branch, she pulled herself into the canopy and continued to climb. She knew that if she could get to the other tree, the cat was too large to follow.

In the next instant, white hot bolts of pain shot through her lower right leg as the Long Tooth's fore claws grazed her. A'nath'a shrieked at the searing sensation but her limbs propelled her further up the tree. She reached again and pulled herself up into the safety of the branches of the other tree.

Deftly maneuvering herself around, oblivious to her wounds, she looked straight into the eyes of the cat as it pulled itself closer, crawling into the branches of the split tree. Her eyes widened further in horror as she slid haltingly back on the branch; surely it couldn't get to her!

As if in response, the branches supporting the cat began to crack. With several loud reports and a roar of frustration, the branches and the cat plummeted as one to the forest floor below, landing with a dull thud and several loud, cracking sounds.

A'nath'a watched, panting heavily, as the cat lay motionless among the shattered branches. Was it dead? After a few moments, slowly, painfully, the Long Tooth began to stir.

One limb at a time, it pulled itself erect, losing its balance momentarily as its left rear leg briefly gave way. The cat looked up at A'nath'a and growled, but it was more a recognition of the situation than a threat. Favoring its uninjured leg, the cat limped slowly into the undergrowth of the forest and, within a few handfuls of heartbeats, disappeared.

Drawing a deep, shuddering breath, A'nath'a quickly assessed her situation. The pain of her leg wounds had turned to a dull throb, but otherwise she was all right. Remembering she had gathered the root for blood sickness, she quickly reached into her sack, still slung around her shoulder, pulled out the root and began to chew it. She grimaced at the bitter taste but knew, more than anyone else in the clan, that it would prevent infection in her wounds. She also knew she was overdue at the cave, and that the clan would soon be looking for her.

She continued to take deep breaths, feeling her racing heart beginning to slow. Scanning quickly across to the lightning-split tree, she found a path which, if she descended carefully, would allow her to safely reach the ground.

Slowly and deliberately, she started to climb back down, carefully testing each branch with her weight as she moved. For one harrowing moment, she teetered precariously on the branch she had chosen, unsure it would support her weight. Thankfully, the branch did not give way and she was easily able to continue over to the shattered trunk of the split tree.

As she began the last phase of her climb down, she heard faint voices, calling her name. With a smile, she returned the calls with her own. They had been looking for her!

As she reached the ground, a party of the clan's males appeared further up the trail. She smiled again as she saw Daorth among them, concern furrowing his brow. As she limped toward them, A'nath'a knew her narrow escape would make a good tale-telling around the fire tonight. Yes, it would be a good evening meal after all!

What A'nath'a Teaches Us. How much of that story can you relate to? While none of us have ever been chased through the forest by a saber tooth cat, all of us have experienced our ancient ancestor A'nath'a's reactions to stress.

In most cases, the Long Tooth is replaced by an angry boss, a dash to the bus, stopping short behind the car in front of you, or a presentation before a judgmental client. Our bodies, however, react in the same way as our primordial ancestor's did. The important difference, however, is that in our case, our lives are usually not actually threatened.

But what exactly did A'nath'a (and we) experience, physiologically? As mentioned earlier, the function of virtually every system in the body is either transformed or modified to respond to the threat. The effects of the stress response therefore include:

- *The blood flow to our brain is radically shifted.* Flow to the portions of the brain that govern the higher mental functions (creativity, judgment, decision making) is constricted. Conversely, flow to the more primitive portion of the brain, which govern reflexes, reaction time, etc., is greatly increased to facilitate either fighting or fleeing.
- *Our senses become more acute.* The pupils of our eyes dilate (enlarge) so we can see more clearly, even in darkness. Our hairs stand on end, making us more sensitive to our environment (and also making us appear larger, hopefully intimidating our opponent). Even our senses of smell and touch become more acute.
- *Our circulatory system goes into overdrive.* Our heart rate accelerates such that our blood flow is increased by up to 500 per cent. Our arteries constrict in order to increase both the overall system pressure and the speed at which blood is delivered to the muscles. The veins expand to facilitate the return of blood to the heart. Sympathetic nervous output tends to divert blood flow

to the large muscles. The body 'thinks' it has to run away from something or fight something and blood flow is correspondingly less to the bowel and other non-muscle organs.

- At the same time, *the smaller blood vessels in our body constrict*, so that any wounds we suffer will not cause excessive blood loss.
- *The lungs, throat and nostrils open up and breathing speeds up* to get more air in the system so the increased blood flow can be re-oxygenated. The blood carries oxygen to the muscles, allowing them to work harder. Deeper breathing also helps us to scream more loudly!
- *The function of the thyroid gland is also temporarily decreased.* Since the stress response is the body's 'overdrive' mechanism, the normal metabolic processes are bypassed.
- *Fat from fatty cells and glucose from the liver are released into the bloodstream* to be used by the muscles for instant energy.
- *The pancreas secretes insulin and enzymes* to allow the glucose to enter and be used by the cells.
- *The raw material for making the adrenal and reproductive hormones, cholesterol and pregnenolone, is diverted primarily to the synthesis of the adrenal hormones.* This also stands to reason: if you're under attack, the last thing you'll be thinking about is reproducing!
- *Blood vessels to the kidney and digestive system constrict.* This shuts down the digestive and elimination systems; they are not immediately essential for escaping the threat. A part of this effect is reduction of saliva in the mouth. This also stands to reason: if we're 'fighting the saber tooth,' we're not going to worry about eating!
- *In extreme cases, the bowels and bladder may release* to reduce the need for expending energy on other internal functions. This might also dissuade our attackers!
- *Sweat glands also open*, providing an external cooling liquid to our over-worked system. This is what makes the skin look pale and clammy.

- *Endorphins, which are the body's natural pain killers, are released.* When you are fighting, you do not want be bothered with pain-that can be put off until later.

These are the most noticeable and significant aspects of the stress response. There are, of course, many others which are not immediately visible to us. But perhaps the most important idea to note is that *this is not a balanced condition in the body!* We can operate this way, in some cases for extended periods, but it is definitely not "homeostasis." The stress response is an adaptive mechanism, where the body operates *out of balance.*

The common element which ties them together, however, and is most important to remember is that *the ability of the body to fuel this response is FINITE.* We do not have the ability to live like this indefinitely. Once again, Rev. Wayne Muller beautifully places this into context:

"When we live without listening to the timing of things – when we live and work in twenty-four hour shifts without rest – we are on war time, mobilized for battle. Yes, we are strong and capable people, we can work without stopping, faster and faster, electric lights making artificial day so the whole machine can labor without ceasing. But remember: no living thing lives like this."

A useful analogy to clarify your understanding of this concept is your company's account at its bank. As long as the company uses its resources effectively, it has the ability to function, even during a short-lived crisis. However, when the company exhausts these financial reserves, its ability to operate ceases shortly thereafter.

Just as your company has a finite account balance from which it can withdraw money, so, too, does our body have a finite ability to respond to stress. As long as the stress response is infrequently activated, our body can respond effectively and, equally important, recuperate from the experience. In many ways, recovery from a stressful experience is like depositing money back into your bank account to replace what you've withdrawn.

However, when the body is repeatedly asked to respond to stressor after stressor, it eventually exhausts the finite bank of energy available to the body. Thus, it only stands to reason that attempting to continually overdraw this bank by chronically overstressing the body will have serious negative health consequences.

Unfortunately, this portion of our body has not evolved at a rate that allows us to use it with the frequency we would like to in our 21st century society. In this respect, we are still more like our ancient ancestors than we would like to admit or believe. Far too many of life's non-life threatening stresses trigger this response.

As a result, the everyday events of contemporary living can leave us in a permanent state of arousal that takes its toll on our bodies. Our modern lifestyle tends to cause continual sympathetic nervous system activation with very little opportunity for the parasympathetic (also called 'vegetative,' or calming) nervous system to activate.

When this parasympathetic system is active, the bowel and other non-muscle organs receive good blood-flow, the pupils constrict, the glands all function well and secrete their various compounds. Absence of parasympathetic activation leads to poor digestion and probably also to poor healing and organ function.

It also happens when a creative new idea makes us feel uncertain about things of which we previously were sure. The biochemical changes in our brain make us aggressive, fighting the new idea, or makes us timid, fleeing from it. This phenomenon was the genesis for Robert M. Sapolksy's aptly named book: *Why Zebras Don't Get Ulcers*.

Stress and the General Adaptation Syndrome (GAS). Doctors call the body's chronic reaction to stress General Adaptation Syndrome (GAS), first described in 1936 by Hans Selye in the journal *Nature*. Selye was able to separate the biological effects of stress from other physical symptoms suffered by patients through his research. He observed that patients suffered physical effects not caused directly by their disease or by their medical condition.

As mentioned earlier, Selye also made the distinction between two specific types of stress: eustress ('positive stress') and distress ('negative stress'), roughly meaning challenge and overload. Both types may be the result of negative or positive events. If a person both gets married and gets fired from his job on the same day, one event does not cancel the other — both are stressful events. What causes distress for one person may cause eustress for another, depending upon each individual's life perception. That reinforces the importance of the influence of the Cognitive Filter. Typically, though, when the word stress is used alone, it is referring to distress.

Selye identified three stages to GAS. In the first stage, called the alarm reaction, the body releases adrenaline and activates a variety of other psychological mechanisms to combat the stress and to stay in control. This is called the fight-or-flight response, and was illustrated and described in detail earlier. When our bodies enter this phase, a key change is the elevation of the important adrenal hormones. When we allow our bodies to return to normal, the levels of these hormones normalize, too. But what if that doesn't happen? If the cause for the stress is not removed, GAS goes to its second stage called *resistance or adaptation*. This is the body's response if it senses the need to provide long-term protection. It secretes further hormones that increase blood sugar levels to sustain energy and raise blood pressure.

Initially, the body is able to maintain the elevated levels of the adrenal hormones. As the stress continues unabated, the adrenal glands will actually increase in size as the body attempts to adjust to the new situation. The medical community calls this condition "*hyperadrenalism*." The adrenals can sometimes grow to *three times* their normal size to attempt to meet the body's demands.

Put that into perspective for yourself: hold up your thumb and look at it. Your adrenals are normally each about the size of that thumb. Now, imagine what your thumb would look like on your hand if it was *three times* its normal size! That's how large your adrenals can grow on top of your kidneys as a chronic stress response continues.

Overuse by the body's defense mechanism in this phase eventually leads to disease. If this adaptation phase continues for a prolonged period of time without periods of relaxation and rest to counterbalance the stress response, sufferers become prone to fatigue, concentration lapses, irritability and lethargy as the effort to sustain arousal slides into negative stress.

This is but one example of what the resistance phase does to the body. Think of your adrenals like the body of a sprinter at a track and field meet: his/her body is bulked up to be able to produce that explosive burst of speed; that's the kind of scenario the now-enlarged adrenals have grown to deal with.

Eventually, though, the demands of the now-chronic stress will overwhelm the body's ability to produce adequate amounts of adrenal hormones, and the production of all will start to diminish. Remember, the body will *always* support the fight-or-flight response before anything else. This process will start to have a slowly increasing, negative impact on all the functions that cortisol, DHEA and aldosterone perform in the body. It is significant and regrettable to note that many people in this country live in this phase of the stress response *their entire lives*.

What are the manifestations that accompany the resistance phase? Keep in mind that everyone has their own unique reaction to stress, and that they may experience some of these manifestations but not others. I've listed a few of the most significant ones below:

Allergies (food, airborne and chemical). The fight-or-flight response redirects a large portion of the immune system's function to the periphery of the body to help protect it against wounding. Since we are dealing with a system of finite resources, it stands to reason that the immune system is now less capable of defending against other threats. An early manifestation of a chronic stress pattern is development of previously undetected allergies or sensitivities to food and chemicals, or aggravated reaction to already existing allergies and sensitivities.

"*Being alone*." We've all experienced the feeling of having to face a major challenge of some sort completely unassisted. Perhaps it was coming to bat in a baseball game as a child with the outcome of the game dependent on your performance; maybe it was getting a loved one to a hospital by yourself during an emergency; or perhaps it was that big sales presentation that would make or break getting the big account. Regardless, under those kinds of stress, you always feel alone.

In his landmark book, *The Biology of Transcendence* (listed in the Resource section) Joseph Chilton Pearce masterfully describes the various functions of the human brain. In particular, he points out that the higher mental functions, such as creativity, judgment, decision making and access to the spiritual, require optimal operation of the pre-frontal cortex, the most advanced part of our brains. In contrast, the so-called 'primitive' parts of our brain, having to do with maintenance of critical autonomic functions and survival reflexes (AKA the stress response), can kick in virtually automatically with the appropriate stimulus.

The body was designed to react and respond effectively to these stimuli on an infrequent, episodic basis in order to escape from threats to its survival. However, 21st Century society has created an environment where the body detects almost constant threats. This has the physiological effect of simultaneously stimulating the 'fight-or-flight' reflex in the more primitive areas of the brain almost constantly while decreasing the blood flow to those areas governing the higher functions.

It is these higher functions that allow us to maintain our sense of connectivity to those people, organizations and spiritual resources that help us to define who we are and to function effectively. By minimizing our ability to access those functions, chronic stress can create the feeling that we are very much alone, and that sense of isolation can lead to the development of psychosomatic disorders such as depression.

Constipation and indigestion. This one should be pretty simple to understand. Under conditions of chronic stress, the body doesn't want to expend energy on anything but survival. That includes digestion and elimination. The longer the stress response lasts, the longer will be the indigestion and constipation.

Dark semi-circles under eyes. The exact sign to look for is a dark quarter circle underneath the inner part of the eye (a full semicircle that extends to the outer part of the eye is an indication that there is some kidney stress involved, as well). This darkness is an early and persistent sign of adrenal stress, a reliable indicator that the body is overtaxing itself.

Decreased libido, increased PMS, and infertility. This is perhaps the classic example of how the body manages its collective energy resources during the fight-or-flight response. Just as the body doesn't want to digest food or eliminate waste under stress, it doesn't want to reproduce, either.

Recall from our earlier discussion that the hormones cortisol, DHEA, aldosterone and the reproductive hormones are all made from the pre-hormonal substance pregnenolone, which in turn is synthesized from cholesterol made by the liver. As the stress response continues, the adrenals will literally steal the pregnenolone from the reproductive organs so that it can sustain the fight-or-flight response. Datis Kharrazian, DC calls this, very aptly, "*pregnenolone steal.*"

Think about that for a minute: how likely will it now be that a woman would be able to enjoy a normal menstrual cycle if her body is not producing enough of any reproductive hormone? If she can't experience a normal menstrual cycle, how likely will it be that she can successfully conceive a child? How likely will it be for a man to have a normal sexual response? These manifestations will continue and worsen if the body is allowed to regress into the exhaustion phase. In an upcoming chapter on the gender-specific effects of chronic stress, we will examine this situation in much greater detail.

Eyes sensitive to bright lights. Recall from A'nath'a's story that her eyes widened (i.e., her pupils dilated) when she confronted the saber tooth. That was to allow more light in and help increase her short term visual acuity. If this situation is allowed to remain unchanged, the above mentioned sensitivity to bright lights can result, as well as an actual *decrease* in visual acuity over time. In other words, chronic stress can contribute to your eventually having to wear glasses!

Grinding teeth, nail biting. I'm sure you can easily figure this one out. With all of the body's responses 'revved up,' and no easily accessible outlet to normalize them, it will try its best to do *something* to remedy the situation. These two manifestations are the most prevalent and easily recognizable.

Headaches. Remember from the first section of the book how the blood flow patterns in the brain changed when A'nath'a was under stress? If those blood flow patterns quickly return to normal, there usually is no headache. However, under chronic stress, the blood vessels at the back of the head remain dilated, giving rise to the well-known 'tension headache.'

Inability to fall asleep. Because the body is stuck in a fight-or-flight response pattern, the adrenal hormones remain elevated, causing the body to continue to be on alert. Let's use an analogy most people are familiar with: night driving. If we have to drive late at night, what do we usually do in order to stay awake? Consume caffeine! We learned earlier that caffeine elevates all the adrenal hormones and puts our body directly into a fight-or-flight response. In the resistance phase of chronic stress, our adrenal hormones remain elevated, just as if we had consumed a cup of coffee. This helps explain why sleep medications are among the top selling pharmaceuticals in this country today.

Increased or lost appetite. How could we experience both? It depends upon where on the stress response scale you are. During the initial "alarm phase," the body doesn't want to deal with anything but escaping the threat, including eating. So it is very likely you could actually lose your appetite (and perhaps a few pounds) as the stress scenario unfolds. However, the body's constant demands for more glucose during the resistance and exhaustion phases eventually cause it to *crave* sugary foods.

Less focused, fuzzier thinking; speech difficulties. Remember that the stress response actually changes the blood flow patterns of the brain, away from the higher mental functions and toward the parts of the brain having to do with the fight-or-flight response. As a result, with the continuance of the chronic stress response it becomes more and more challenging for us to access those higher mental functions, including memory access and speech.

A 'can't miss' manifestation of this phenomenon in action is when you consistently have trouble accessing information such as names of people, work-related data, or you consistently trip over words and phrases. One of my most interesting and enjoyable teachers, Dr. I. Michael Borkin, NMD, likens this to taking a file cabinet and dumping all its files on the floor. If you are then asked to find a file folder, you have to go through all the files in order to find it. The brain under stress works in much the same way; in this 'files on the floor' condition, the information is there, but it's disorganized and increasingly difficult to access.

Lower back pain. Recall that the adrenals sit on top of the kidneys, right below the bottom of the rear rib cage. Persistent pain in this area can be an important indicator of chronic stress.

Muscle aches. Earlier in the book, we identified the adrenal hormone cortisol as playing an important part in the relief of pain and inflammation during the fight-or-flight response. Make no mistake; when A'nath'a was wounded by the saber tooth, her cortisol was flowing! But if we are stuck in this same pattern, we gradually become less able to counteract the accompanying inflammation. Result: muscle aches.

Non-specific joint pain/arthritis. This was one of my most fascinating discoveries during my study and research, again thanks to Dr. Borkin. You'll remember from earlier in this chapter that the stress response causes the hypothalamus to direct the adrenal medulla to secrete the hormones epinephrine and norepinephrine, which help modulate the central nervous system portion of the stress response. They are delivered into the bloodstream in the form of microscopic crystalline shards. If used to assist with the stress response, no problem.

However, if not used, just like glucose they are stored in the body. Any ideas where? How about the synovial fluid of the joints! Dr. Borkin asserts that about 80 per cent of the arthritis diagnoses in this country are actually this reaction to the unfulfilled fight-or-flight response.

The validity of this assertion was driven home to me with one of my very first clients. Rose was a flight attendant I had flown with who came to me with a variety of stress-related complaints; prominent among them was persistent knee pain of a degree that caused her to seriously consider surgery. After we worked a couple of weeks to help her detoxify her body, the pain was gone. She called it *"the cheapest knee surgery I've ever heard of."*

Psychosomatic changes (more impatient, mild depression, less enjoyment/happiness with life). As the biochemical changes in the brain under stress continue, the emphasis on the efficient operation of the part that controls the stress response will increase, as will the deemphasis on the brain's higher functions. This includes those parts of the brain controlling emotional response. As a result, we begin to operate in a state called 'decreased emotional margin.' This is a condition where events and stimuli which cause an unstressed person virtually no concern will precipitate an emotional overreaction. Occurring either simultaneously or separately will be episodes of mild depression, also tied intimately to the brain's changing functional state.

The third stage of GAS is called exhaustion. In this stage, the body has run out of its reserve of body energy and immunity. Because of the significance of its manifestations, as well as its prevalence among our fellow Americans, we'll talk about the exhaustion phase in much more detail in the following chapter.

About the time of the publication of Selye's initial research findings, the gradual realization dawned that descriptions of conditions such as anxiety, antagonism, exhaustion, frustration, distress, despair, overwork, pre-menstrual tension, over-focusing, confusion, mourning and fear could all be incorporated into a broader definition of the term stress. The popular use of the term as it applied to these conditions expanded rapidly. The ultimate result was the creation of an entire industry of stress management, encompassing the fields of popular psychology, self-help, and personal counseling.

As we have seen earlier, any factor that creates a stress response in the body is called a stressor. While we have already derived several categories in the Stress Stack, it is useful for us to examine other categorizations as well. For example, many researchers contend there are two kinds of stressors: processive stressors and systemic stressors.

Processive stressors are elements in the environment (for example, elevated sound levels or bright light) perceived by the organism as potential dangers. These do not cause damage directly, but are processed in the cerebral cortex. The processed information is then sent via the limbic system in the hypothalamus, where they activate the supreme centers of the autonomic nervous system. This results in the fight-or-flight (or sympathetico-adrenal) response. Examples of this kind of stressor can be found in the Lifestyle Influences, Cognitive Filter or Trigger Factor blocks of the Stress Stack.

Systemic stressors, on the other hand, cause a disturbance in the organism's homeostasis, as well as tissue death in the body, hypotension (low blood pressure) and/or hypoxia (low oxygen in the tissues of the organism). Often both types of stressors occur simultaneously. They are usually accompanied by pain and/or intense emotions. Examples of this type of stressor can be found in the Dietary Influences, Nutritional Gap, and Toxic Influences blocks of the Stress Stack.

How It All Works. Researchers now believe that the neurochemistry of the general adaptation syndrome is well understood. However, much remains to be discovered about how this system interacts with other systems in the brain and elsewhere in the body.

In summary, the body reacts to stress first by releasing two types of hormones: the catecholamine hormones, epinephrine (otherwise known as adrenaline) and norepinephrine; and the glucocorticoid hormones, primarily cortisol, DHEA and aldosterone. The catecholamine hormones are primarily associated with the activation of the central nervous system and control of blood pressure. The glucocorticoid hormones are associated with the emergency activation of the body's energy production processes and control of inflammation, although aldosterone does play an important role in blood pressure regulation.

The hypothalamic-pituitary-adrenal (HPA) axis is a major part of the neuroendocrine system, involving the interactions of the hypothalamus and pituitary glands (the 'front office') and the adrenal glands (the 'crisis management department'). The HPA axis plays a primary role in the body's reactions to stress. It balances the release of both the catecholamine and glucocorticoid hormones.

The use of the term stress in serious recognized conditions such as those of post-traumatic stress disorder and psychosomatic illness has, unfortunately, somewhat blurred the analysis of the generalized 'stress' phenomenon. Regardless, stress resulting from negative life events, or distress, and from positive life events, or eustress, can clearly have a serious physical impact distinct from the situations experienced by most people, whom psychotherapists call the 'worried well.' The Stress Stack offers you a description of the major categories of these life events and influences.

What Happens If. . .?   So far, we've looked at the operation of 'The Endocrine Co.' during the initial crisis stage (alarm reaction) and the adaptation (resistance) phase. But what happens when we go beyond those stages, when we ignore Lin Yutang's advice and dismiss the importance of discovering what we *can't* do?   What happens when we ask the 'head of the spider' to keep us in overdrive? What occurs when, as frequently happens in our society, we 'strip our gears' and almost literally burn ourselves out? Turn the page to find the answer!

CHAPTER 5

EFFECTS OF CHRONIC STRESS:
BREAKING THE BANK

"Under the biochemical influence of [chronic stress], the body concludes that stress is always going to be present and stops trying to restore balance. Blood pressure, heart rate, and cortisol levels remain elevated. What was meant to be a temporary emergency state becomes a way of life where the pleasures of deep relaxation, peace, and tranquility are no longer available."

— Stephen Cherniske, M.S., "Caffeine Blues"

Overdrawing Your Account: the Setup. So far, we have looked at several important aspects of stress and the effects of the *normal* stress response. We have seen that some stressors, e.g., moderate regular exercise, can actually be healthful. The recognized worldwide pioneer in the arena of stress research, Hans Selye MD, called this type of stress 'eustress,' or good stress. But what about the other kind of stress, the kind Selye called 'distress?' It is *this* type of stress that generated the title of this work, and is at the root of so much of the ill health that afflicts Corporate America, and our society at large, today.

As many of you might expect, most of my clientele come to see me after they have been 'around the block and back again' with the conventional health care community. J.S. was just such a person; her story is a perfect example of the effects of Dr. Selye's 'distress.'

She happened on a magazine article I had written after she had been to her second medical hormone balancing clinic in a year. Her level of frustration at the lack of success was exacerbated when, having completed the second clinic's protocol with no meaningful improvement, she asked the doctor running the clinic what the next step was. The response: "*I don't know.*"

Her out-of-pocket expenses by this time were in the thousands of dollars (neither of these clinics accepted insurance for most of their treatment programs). Her description of her own condition was simple: "*I'm falling apart, and I don't know what to do about it.*" She complained about her 'zero' energy level, indigestion and constipation, poor quality sleep with virtually no energy when she awakened and, most important, her inability to do even the simplest tasks without feeling physically, mentally and emotionally overwhelmed.

To understand the magnitude of the impact of this type of 'distress,' recall the characteristics of the normal stress response we discussed in the previous chapter. Specifically, the normal stress response characteristics: *are designed for brief, intense response* (such as 'fleeing/fighting the saber tooth' like our prehistoric ancestor A'nath'a did); *require specific physical activity* to normalize the body once the response is activated (again, A'nath'a physically, aerobically exerted herself to both flee the threat and normalize her body's responses); *exert a cumulative effect on the body* if the response is not normalized (in other words, 'a couple of weeks off' won't suffice!); are systemic, affecting virtually every bodily system (literally, like dropping a pebble in a pond); *are physiologically supportive for only a short time* (the opposite, chronic response is therefore destructive over time); *when allowed to degenerate into a chronic pattern, set the stage for serious physiological breakdown.*

J.S.' situation is a textbook description of the latter: degeneration into a chronic stress pattern leading to exhaustion. In her case, and that of so many others, her stress response had been activated far beyond the resistance phase described by Hans Selye. She was deep into the exhaustion phase of General Adaptation Syndrome (GAS), her body teetering on the brink of serious illness.

In this stage, the body has run out of its reserves of bodily energy and immune response. The 'bank account' has been almost completely depleted. Mental, physical and emotional reserves are almost at their end. As the adrenals become depleted, the person experiences decreased stress tolerance and progressive mental and physical exhaustion, leading in most cases to illness and collapse.

In order to fully understand J.S.' regression to this regrettable situation, please first recall my discussion in Chapter 1 about a phenomenon called the 'catabolic threshold.' As applied to stress management, it is the accumulation of stressors which push our bodies' stress response into the zone where destructive changes to our organ systems begin to take place, resulting in the onset of disease.

How does this happen? As we saw early in Chapter 1, there are almost as many definitions of stress as there are people. Many factors contribute to a catabolic stress response, and the mixture of each is different with every person. To help simplify things and increase your understanding, I developed the six blocks of the Stress Stack. Factors in all six of these blocks contribute in one way or another to creating the exhaustion phase in our bodies.

Dietary Influences: The Bank Account Is Nearly Empty. We talked at length about the most significant of these, caffeine, artificial sweeteners, processed sugar, white flour and trans fats, in Chapters 1 and 3. Unfortunately, these are the 'quick fixes' that most people reach for when attempting to cope with stress. While perhaps temporarily satisfying a need for 'more energy,' the practical effect is that they each either directly or indirectly activate the fight-or-flight response. In reality, they actually make your body *less* able to generate the right kind of energy production and add to the problem of exhaustion even more.

In the case of caffeinated foods or beverages, the response is direct: consume caffeine, and your body goes into fight-or-flight. The response is a bit more complicated when the other foods are ingested, but the practical result is the same: an increase in the body's stress response.

If you were to boil the process down to its simplest explanation, it would be '*drink a cup of coffee, eat a candy bar or bagel, or drink a diet soda, and your body reacts, in whole or in part, as if you're being chased by the saber tooth.*'

However, once the body enters the exhaustion phase, it doesn't possess the energy reserves to produce the right kinds of adrenal hormones at the right times and in the right quantities. Although the demand for the body to respond to the stressor(s) is there, the supply of energy isn't.

It's not unusual for people like this to start experiencing weight gain, chest pains, heart palpitations, and extreme exhaustion. Continuing to use these foods and beverages to attempt to sustain yourself spirals you deeper and more rapidly into ever increasing exhaustion.

Lifestyle Influences: Your Bank Balance Shows An Overdraft. Recall that there are a myriad of lifestyle influences that impact the body's stress response. They include such factors as chronic inadequate sleep, unalleviated stress at the workplace or at home, toxic relationships, and stress-causing activities such as over exercising or chronic use of suspenseful video games. Let's look a little closer at each of these in turn.

If there is one stress factor that is almost universal in this country today, it is the chronic lack of sleep that afflicts most Americans. Go to any office, school, place of business or government agency and you'll see the evidence for yourself. We talked earlier about some of the factors impacting this problem, but there is definitely more to discuss.

For as long as there has been a health care system in this country, there have been repeated calls by its leadership for 'at least seven to eight hours of sleep a night.' At the beginning of the last century, achieving that goal was not a hard thing to do. After all, the majority of the population of this country still lived in a largely rural environment. There were few activities after dark to distract one from getting a good night's sleep. Widespread air travel was decades away; chronic interruption of one's circadian rhythm was virtually unheard of.

A humorous story related by my mother about her high school years highlights the lighting conditions that existed at that time. She and my aunt were double dating, riding in the convertible Model T belonging to one of their dates, when they passed through a grove of trees on their way home. In the darkness (there were no streetlights out in the country back then), they did not see a small screech owl light in my aunt's hair. Only when they re-entered the moonlight on the other side of the grove did they see the creature perched on my aunt's head. To put this episode in context, it was unusual for people who lived in the country to be out after dark, so there was no need for extensive road lighting systems at that time.

After World War II, however, the combination of the wholesale migration of the population from farm to city, unprecedented economic growth, and technological innovation created an environment where adequate sleep rapidly became, and remains, an elusive goal for an ever increasing number of Americans. While we all marvel at the safety enhancements that now allow us to travel in relative security in any part of the country at virtually any hour, and at the myriad of entertainment options which are available to us 24/7, the price we pay is an ever increasing deficit of adequate sleep.

Although some segments of society lead to us believe (another 'hypnosis') that this doesn't have an effect on our ability to function as productive members of society, the data says otherwise. Chronic lack of sleep results in systemic decreases in organ system efficiency, decreased productivity at home, work and school, increased susceptibility to accidents, and reliance on the 'usual suspects' of caffeinated beverages and sugar to 'get us through the day.'

Why does lack of sleep affect us this way? The explanation delves into some of the most complex interactions of the brain and body, a detailed explanation of which would comprise an entire book itself. However, two important points must be addressed in order for us to clearly appreciate the need for adequate sleep.

The first is that, while sleeping, the body experiences cycles of approximately ninety minutes. During each cycle it moves through all the different stages of sleep, including the best known, rapid eye movement (REM), associated with the dream state. Mark Stibich, PhD, a behavioral change expert, offers an easily understandable explanation of each of these phases. Stage 1, light sleep, is the one from which you can most easily be awakened. This ease of awakening highlights the importance of having a favorable sleep environment (i.e., a dark, quiet room with a comfortable temperature). Stage 2, which comprises about half of your total night's sleep, is the transition phase to deeper sleep, when your brain waves slow and eye movement stops. Stage 3, the initial stage of deep sleep, and stage 4, the secondary stage of deep sleep, are the two from which it is most difficult to awaken someone. Both stages are needed to provide refreshing sleep. Finally, REM, the stage where dreaming occurs, comprises about one fifth of sleep for adults. Research has shown that REM sleep is critical for the development of long-term memory. However, it is important to note that *all* of the stages of sleep are interconnected and important for the body to receive adequate rest.

At the same time these stages of sleep are occurring, another more significant, 8 hour cycle is taking place. During the first four hours, the body is mobilizing its repair and reconstitution resources to address the *physical* rejuvenation and repair needs of the body. During the second four hours, the focus is on the repair of the *psychological and emotional* functions. This part of the cycle allows us to subconsciously address and come to terms with the stressors of the previous day, as well as to delve into some of the deeper emotional issues which can only be safely and effectively addressed in deep sleep.

Thus, we can easily see that we all need to move through at least five of the shorter cycles, and both parts of the longer, 8 hour cycle to obtain meaningful, healthful, adequate rest. Doing less will subject us to the effects of one or more types of chronic sleep deficit: either we will shortchange our psychological repair mechanisms and allow the progressive deterioration of our mental and emotional states or, if the sleep deficit is even more severe, start the chain of catabolic processes which result in the deterioration of our physical health and descent into chronic illness.

Perhaps the most dramatic example of the effects of chronic sleep deprivation can be found in the experience of combat troops. Exposed continually to the very high stress environment of battle, they usually are able to manage only a few hours' sleep each night, only to awaken and repeatedly re-insert themselves into the same stress-laden environment. Over time, this pattern of deprivation robs them of the psychological and then physical recuperation necessary to sustain their mental, emotional and physical well being.

It's no wonder these troops return from combat duty with a variety of psychological and physical ailments, the most prevalent being post-traumatic stress disorder (PTSD).

Sleep deprivation is a major contributing lifestyle factor to descent into the exhaustion phase of a chronic stress response. Unfortunately, the very thing the body needs most to enjoy a good night's sleep, a normal stress hormonal cycle, is unavailable to people in this exhausted state. A map of the secretion of the adrenal hormone cortisol for someone experiencing this level of exhaustion would look like a straight horizontal line at the bottom of the measuring scale, indicating little to no hormonal secretion.

In this state, the body is so depleted that it is unable to produce the right amounts of adrenal hormones at the right time to allow it to rest, recuperate and rebuild. The result is that a person will typically wake up continually throughout the night, getting at most a few hours rest, and awaken in the morning feeling as if they haven't slept at all.

There are many strategies which sleep experts have devised to describe both the sleep deficit 'hole' we are digging for ourselves and the means to overcome it. The common element they all have is that you can't make up for lost sleep by simply 'sleeping in' on the weekend. As a practical matter, by the time you reach the point where you feel you have to do that in order to face the week ahead, you're already well down the road to both exhaustion and a catabolic stress response. That's because *chronic stress increases the rate at which we age, and decreases the age at which we die.*

Recall in the Preface that I identified the New York City area as *"one of the highest stress environments in the country."* Some Big Apple dwellers would probably take strong exception to that statement, but it is a truism. Unalleviated stress in the workplace and at home were two primary factors in the demise of my parents and their contemporaries, even though at the time neither they nor I were cognizant of the destructive processes at work in their lives. By destructive, I mean that the cumulative load of the demands of responding effectively in the workplace and at home take an increasing toll if they outstrip the ability of the body to cope (there's that word *cumulative* again!).

A classic example of this phenomenon in action walked up to our booth one afternoon at an expo devoted to women's life and health issues. Della was a personable, attractive woman in her late forties. A middle school teacher, she proceeded at a rapid fire pace to relate a dizzying tale of all of the stressors being inflicted upon her, especially the twin demands of employment and child-rearing responsibilities.

She then proceeded to relate an even more dizzying array of manifestations which her frenetic lifestyle had wrought on her health: mood swings, weight gain, that 'falling apart' feeling, digestive issues, hot flashes, poor sleep, and a dozen more. After she read our displays and literature, she made an appointment to see me on the spot.

A week later, citing the incredible demands her children's activities placed on her, she cancelled, promising to reschedule 'sometime in the summer.' Sadly, we have yet to hear from her. Della's situation and countless more like hers are what is unfortunately becoming the norm, not only in Corporate America, but in society at large.

The subject of relationships and their effect on your physical, mental and emotional health is one which has been analyzed, dissected, and discussed at great length in a very large number of books. We touched on it briefly in an earlier chapter. As such, we will not attempt to turn this portion of the book into another personal prescription for supportive and fulfilling relationships.

Instead, please be clearly aware that while supportive relationships can be an incredible boon in dealing with chronic stress, toxic relationships can be as destructive stressors as any of the other factors I will mention. By toxic, I mean those relationships which do not leave you feeling supported, nurtured, encouraged or respected (depending who you are relating to). Toxic relationships can surface in the home, school, workplace or virtually anywhere.

As mentioned earlier, we have all had the experience of knowing someone who 'pushes our buttons,' i.e., who because of their own psychological and emotional makeup, and their relationship to us, knows exactly how to access the part of us that causes us to react in a certain way. If the 'buttons' they push are positive, then the relationship experience can be very supportive and uplifting. However, if the 'buttons,' either intentionally or unintentionally, unlock old emotional wounds or are overtly disrespectful and/or abusive, and are pushed on a continuing basis, they are part of the toxic relationships which add to our stress load, pushing us ever closer to the exhaustion phase of the stress response.

One way in which many people attempt to cope with stress is through exercise. That is certainly one of the most healthful means by which we can manage stress. However, since the early 1980s, the fitness craze has spawned a new type of stressor which has become a major contributor to our level of chronic stress: over exercising.

By that, I mean continuous, strenuous, almost daily exercise to the point of physical exhaustion. Why would someone expose their bodies to such extensive physical abuse? In a word: endorphins. These are chemical substances typically produced by the pituitary and hypothalamus which, when released into the bloodstream (by the pituitary) and brain (by the hypothalamus), create the 'feel good' sensation we have all experienced at one time or another in our lives.

Endorphins can be released when we are in love, when we experience an intensely positive response to things such as breathtaking scenery, or when we reach the plateau in intense physical exercise where we feel like we can go on forever. It is the latter scenario, attained on occasion by highly conditioned athletes, which can precipitate a virtual addiction to over exercising.

Many ultra-endurance athletes speak longingly of the 'endorphin pump' they experience during long distance exercise; because of the intensity of the pleasurable feelings, they continually attempt to duplicate the conditions which led to their first experience. This addiction can lead to obsessive, self-destructive behavior.

For example, a health professional I know of suffers from severe knee degeneration due to years of long distance running on asphalt and concrete. Despite the almost constant pain, he still ran many miles per week in an increasingly vain attempt to again experience that 'endorphin pump.'

Additionally, we recently watched with sadness as the Kennedy clan lost another member, this one to over exercising. Kara Kennedy, the late Senator Ted Kennedy's daughter, collapsed and died after a strenuous workout at a health club. While the family admitted that she had been weakened by the treatments for her previously successful battle with lung cancer, the fact remains that she did not respect her own body's limits, with tragic results.

As I'm sure you've figured out by now, there is a definite downside to this type of activity. Recall from Chapter 4 that a major function of the adrenal hormone cortisol is to help control pain and inflammation. Now apply that information to the health professional I discussed above. Is it any wonder that, over time, his adrenals are shot?

A constant application of large amounts of intense stress on his body generates tremendously high levels of inflammation, not only in his joints, muscles and connective tissue, but also in his cardiovascular system. This in turn requires an almost constant demand on his adrenals to attempt to control the resulting inflammation.

While he may believe he is maintaining a high level of fitness, in fact he is breaking down his body just as surely as if he was eating poorly and indulging in destructive health habits like smoking and excessive drinking. This scenario is even more remarkable because, as a health professional, he should know better. The point is that no matter which stressors you inflict on the body, the end result is the same: adrenal exhaustion, and personally experiencing the fact that *chronic stress increases the rate at which we age, and decreases the age at which we die.*

I mentioned briefly in Chapter 3 that stressful video entertainment, from television, movies or video games, can cause a detrimental stress response. To cite a personal example, I recently received an e-mail from a friend of mine who is a very powerful energetic healer. The morning before, she had received a call from a client suffering with cardiovascular disease.

This client, who had previously undergone many types of cardiac treatment, was in a panic, having watched a frightening reality movie alone on late night TV and then spent an exhausting, sleepless night. Talk about cardiac risk factors!

But perhaps the most prevalent example, and the one which holds the most risk for long-term societal dysfunction, is the prevalence of very violent and graphic video games, usually purchased and played by young men. Emerging research has shown that these games cause measurable and detrimental changes in the way the brain operates.

As it applies to the stress response, the part of the brain called the hippocampus, which helps control emotions and the decision making processes, starts to deteriorate when chronically exposed to the adrenal hormone cortisol. This is the same response generated in the body by soldiers in combat, and for them frequently results in the onset of PTSD! Is it any wonder that these games are now believed to decrease the inhibition of the players toward commission of violent acts?

At the same time, many gamers participate in multi-player, online games late into the night. They use caffeine to stay awake, and add both caffeine dependence and chronic sleep deprivation to their health issues. If they then have to face a corporate employment situation the next day, they continue to use caffeine to stay alert (read that: 'wired') throughout he day, their bodies literally hurtling toward adrenal exhaustion and the catabolic threshold.

The Cognitive Filter: The Overdraft Notices Keep Piling Up.
The third block of the Stress Stack, the 'Cognitive Filter,' was also discussed extensively in Chapter 1. Recall that it is the combination of physical, mental, emotional and spiritual factors that collectively create the prism through which we view the world.

Famous authors such as Norman Vincent Peale have for years advocated 'the power of positive thinking,' but as we saw earlier, our thoughts and many other stressors can literally cause the body to create hormones, including adrenal hormones. A chronic pattern of this type of negative behavior sets the body up for a catabolic stress response and ultimately leads to exhaustion.

Although we extensively discussed almost all the components of the cognitive filter in Chapter 1, a crucial one needs to be further addressed here: the importance of one's emotional state. Remember that the cognitive filter changes constantly as a function of the inputs/stimuli it receives. This is especially true when describing the influence of the emotions.

To understand why, imagine that you are driving your car down a mountain dirt road, one that is strewn with rocks, fallen tree branches, and potholes. Now let's imagine that you have to reach an intersection with another road way up ahead, and the only way you can do so is to navigate around those obstacles.

Logic dictates that you will decide which way offers you the least hazardous route around those obstacles and then drive your car over that route. Typically, one of the ways you decide will be to determine if there are ruts in the road that have been worn by people taking a given route before you. If you are successful in navigating around these obstacles, you will likely use the same technique when you reach a point further down the road and encounter similar obstacles. However, the risk you run is that you will ignore 'the road less traveled,' and in the process deny yourself a potentially easier route.

In many ways, the programming your brain undergoes when a stimulus generates a given emotion works much like that. You are, literally, creating a 'rut in the road,' a bit of memory programmed into the brain that you now have available for reference later on. When the memory bit reinforces a valuable or productive reaction, the resulting emotion can be very positive and healthful. However, when the memory bit reinforces a 'rut' that is negative or unhealthful, a stress response results.

This is especially true when the emotion is the result of chronic stressors, such as childhood abuse, illness or serious injury. Sometimes, the 'rut' can become so deep that it obscures access to other, more healthful forms of emotional expression.

This influence is an important contributor to the onset and progression of many serious illnesses, but none more so than cancer. One of the most important lessons I have learned in my practice has been the pivotal influence of the long-term emotional state of a client who has been offered a medical diagnosis of any type of cancer. While we traditional naturopaths don't claim to treat or cure any disease, much less cancer, we do look at the key health imbalances underlying the disease process and help to address those imbalances so the body can effectively take over and finish the job of healing itself.

With respect to cancer, these imbalances include (but are not limited to) an acid constitution (i.e., low pH), poor cellular oxygenation, high free radical count, an ongoing inflammatory process, poor diet (usually characterized by high consumption of sugary foods), and compromised immune system function. In many cases, you can also add to this some sort of toxic influence, which could be chemical, biological or radiological. But underlying all of these is frequently an unhealthful emotional state, in many cases one which has been embedded within the client's thought and emotional processes for years, perhaps even decades, and of which the client may not even be aware.

By the time such clients arrive at my door, they have usually already been through the various stages of the medical treatment system and either been told that they must undergo traumatic, radical therapies (i.e., chemotherapy, radiation and/or surgery) to save their lives or, worse yet, that the disease process is so advanced that nothing more can be done. As you might expect, the predominant, overwhelming emotion expressed by these people is fear.

However, before I agree to work with clients with such a diagnosis, I always ask them two important questions. First, what are your future plans (in other words, do you have any, or have you just resigned yourself to death)? Second, who or what are you distressed about?

The second question, especially, results in the opening of the emotional floodgates for many. Two examples from my case files clearly demonstrate the powerful influence emotion has on the body's stress response and therefore on its state of health.

Mary (not her real name) was brought to me by her daughter, a former client, in hopes that I would be able to help Mary's body better withstand the aggressive radiation and chemotherapy regimen her oncologist had indicated was necessary to save her life. While gathering her health history, two remarkable facts stood out. First, as a stress management technique Mary relied on overeating, primarily processed food products made of white flour. In the complementary and alternative health world, a virtual mantra concerning cancer's internal workings is that 'cancer loves sugar (or glucose, the byproduct of white flour).'

Second, her life history was punctuated by frequent physical, mental and emotional abuse, beginning with her childhood in the northern plains and continuing with her now-long divorced husband. As a result, the other coping strategy Mary learned was to never show an emotional reaction to pain, likely an unfortunate result of her parents' child raising philosophy. Although we attempted to help her address these significant underlying emotional issues, even suggesting she seek professional counseling, she refused.

We attempted to devise a workable strategy for Mary to address all these health concerns in a way she could deal with. However, despite the best supportive efforts of us and her family, the emotional 'ruts in the road' proved too deep. After just a few days, she reverted to her old coping strategies, including both her dysfunctional eating habits and not one expression of discomfort during her painful medical treatments. When last we heard from her family, she was not faring well.

In contrast, you may recall one of the people to whom I have dedicated my book was a remarkable woman by the name of Margie. In contrast to the other case histories, which I have altered out of respect for my clients' privacy, Margie insisted I tell her story. I have changed some details to protect her family's privacy, but the other personal aspects of Margie's story are as she would have wanted me to tell them.

Margie and I first met at a church function that she, my wife and I attended. She was remarkable for a single woman of 75. Despite her previous bout with colon cancer, she exuded an almost unbridled optimism. Though well past 'retirement age,' she was still working full time, actively involved in her church, and enjoying the companionship of a wide circle of friends.

Unfortunately, the first common element Margie shared with Mary was a taste for processed food, in particular white flour products. That, and some of the demands placed upon her at work and at home, led to a recurrence of the colon cancer in a metastatic form. By the time she sought our help in September of 2004, the cancer had spread to her lymph nodes and her medical diagnosis was terminal, offering at best three to six months. It prompted her compassionate internist to courageously (for an MD) recommend that "*maybe the alternative route is the best way for you now.*"

Margie's reaction to my second question, though, was totally unlike Mary's. She reflected on it for a moment, and admitted there were anger-related issues in her life, centering primarily on her family relationships, that she needed to work on. At a later session, she told me that no one had ever before brought that up as a factor in her illness, that it made perfect sense, and that she had made it a priority in her personal spiritual practice (which included daily meditation) to come to terms with it.

From the beginning of our working together, Margie displayed an insatiable curiosity and amazing sense of humor about the whys and wherefores of our remedies and assessment techniques. At one point, while I was performing a bioenergetic assessment on her, she remarked that "*no matter how this all turns out, I find it so interesting!*" You could have knocked me over with a feather.

Although we were able to help stave off the debilitating effects of her health challenge for an additional 15 months, Margie had regrettably crossed the catabolic threshold long before she came to see us, and the result was inevitable. What was remarkable was the effect her coming to terms with her negative emotions had on both the length of time she was able to enjoy quality of life, and the manner in which she was able to make her transition.

Taken into the home of close friends, her last days were spent in a beautiful environment of loving support and spiritual sustenance. Incredibly, though she was obviously wasting away, she reported absolutely no pain, and actually was able to move about by herself until just a few hours before she died.

I had the privilege of being at her bedside about four days before she made her transition. As always, her spirits were up, but she obviously had something she wished to discuss with me. She first asked me that if, in my opinion, she had 'gone the alternative route' at an earlier point, she would have stood a better chance of survival. I told her that I honestly didn't know for sure, but that I had a great deal of confidence in the ability of changing the underlying biological terrain to positively affect virtually any health challenge.

She thought about that for a moment, and then took my hand in hers. "*I want you to promise me that you will continue your healing work (physical and spiritual) after I'm gone. You've helped me so much, and you have a great gift to share with the world. I'll be keeping tabs on you, and I'll be disappointed if you don't keep your promise."* I told her I would keep my promise and, with tears in my eyes, kissed her goodbye on her forehead. She was gone four days later.

I am totally convinced that the additional time she was able to spend on this planet, and the manner of her passing, were primarily, positively and materially affected by her ability to climb out of her own emotional 'ruts in the road' and take a new path. Hers is the most compelling story I can share about the incredible power of the emotions to affect one's health.

At the same time, the experiences of both Margie and Mary portray very starkly the inevitable result if we abuse our bodies and continue to allow the blocks of our Stress Stack to grow. Their situations, and those of countless others who experience the ravages of cancer, sadly make the case for the most important lesson I can again share with you: *chronic stress increases the rate at which we age, and decreases the age at which we die.*

The "Nutritional Gap": No Transfers From Other Accounts. The fourth factor adversely impacting our rate of descent into the exhaustion phase is the 'nutritional gap' that most of us suffer from. Why 'most of us?' The Council for Responsible Nutrition, a Washington DC-based health advocacy group, conducted a survey in 2007 of American's dietary habits. While they found that over 80 per cent of Americans recognized that eating a balanced diet was important, *only 20 per cent of Americans reported actually eating a balanced diet every day!* Keep in mind that that figure was determined by self-reporting, so the actual figure may be somewhat lower; not everyone who claims they eat a balanced diet actually does.

How does that contribute to a descent into the exhaustion phase? It deprives us of the key nutrients that the body needs to sustain a healthy stress response. Several of those key nutrients are in short supply in the Standard American Diet.

For example, the adrenal gland tissues have about 25 times the vitamin C content of the rest of the body's tissues. They use this vitamin C as an integral part of the stress response. As such, when the body is under stress, it also needs a means of replenishing itself after a stressful episode.

Unfortunately, the combination of the lack of meaningful levels of vitamin C in most of the foods we eat, and the depletion of vitamin C by chronic exposure to stressors such as caffeine leaves most of us behind the power curve when it comes to sustaining our vitamin C levels. Keep that up long enough, and you have created a major part of your nutritional gap.

Likewise, the central nervous system uses the B vitamins to sustain its portion of the stress response. The same types of stressors that deplete vitamin C can also detrimentally impact the B vitamin levels in your body. So with the lack of central nervous system support, the gap grows even larger.

Additionally, the raw material the body uses to synthesize the adrenal hormones cortisol, DHEA and aldosterone are made from the nutrients provided by the Omega 3 essential fatty acids, primarily available from cold water fish like salmon and tuna. If someone either doesn't like fish, overreacts to the negative publicity surrounding the mercury content in fish and chooses not to eat it, or doesn't take a good quality Omega 3 supplement, then they deprive their body of the very things they most need to keep adequate amounts of those adrenal hormones available.

Likewise, the body burns through several key minerals, such as magnesium, when it's under stress. If someone is not careful about either including those sources of minerals in their diet, or supplementing with a good quality multi-mineral supplement, they continue to widen their nutritional gap and hasten the arrival of the exhaustion phase.

Toxic Influences: The Outflow Continues to Exceed the Input. The fifth factor is exposure to the large number of toxic materials (i.e., heavy metals, chemicals, radiation, bacteria, viruses, and parasites) with which we all have to contend. Each of these types of toxins has very unique and specific influences on the body. As a group, they add to the stress load we must contend with daily.

As mentioned in Chapter 1, in the last 50 years of man's existence on this planet we have been exposed to more toxic chemicals than in the previous 200,000 years. Of these, by far the most toxic are the heavy metals, such as cadmium, mercury, lead, etc.

In all fairness, when these chemicals were first introduced into products that humans used on a daily basis, no one knew they were harmful. For example, the ancient Romans extensively used lead to construct the pipes of their water delivery systems. An intriguing theory has arisen that a significant factor in the fall of the Roman Empire was the mental lassitude caused by progressive poisoning of the population through lead leaching from the pipes into the water supply. An interesting idea, to be sure. But no ancient Roman scientist, regardless of the advanced nature of his schooling, had the level of knowledge to accurately assess this threat.

The same can be said for both cadmium and mercury. When smoking tobacco was first adopted by Europeans in the New World, in the person of Sir Walter Raleigh, no one knew that the smoke contained extremely harmful deposits of cadmium, one of the most toxic of the heavy metals. And the first dentists to have used mercury amalgams to fill teeth certainly had no idea of the effects of microscopic particles of mercury on the human physiology.

All this data on the toxicity of heavy metals surfaced long after these products were in established use. The challenge facing us today is to find a way to eliminate the influence of each of these toxins in an economically feasible manner. And eliminate them we must, because each of them is a major cause of physiological stress, and chronic exposure to any of them sets the stage for the onset of a variety of serious illnesses. Once again, *chronic stress increases the rate at which we age, and decreases the age at which we die.*

A very similar phenomenon takes place in the chemical arena. The Chapter 1 example of the use of soft plastics for beverage bottling is the most dramatic case I can offer concerning widespread chemical contamination in our society. A chronic exposure of this type results in a long-term stress response, similar in nature to that caused by heavy metals.

The discovery of the existence and application of X-Ray radiation ranks as one of the most important in scientific and medical history. For the first time, doctors were able to noninvasively peer into the human body and gather important information about patients' health concerns. However, as our civilization has continued to advance, the prevalence with which we are being exposed, sometimes unknowingly, to harmful radiation sources has reached alarming levels.

A typical business day for countless corporate employees will expose them to large doses of cell phone radiation, Wi-Fi networks, radiation from computer equipment/monitors and TV screens, and perhaps some sort of security screening device, if they happen to commute to work via subway or train. Add in the occasional airline trip, whose hazards were previously discussed, and we have set in place another source of chronic, cumulative stress which *increases the rate at which we age, and decreases the age at which we die.*

While our advanced civilization has made tremendous strides in the areas of sanitation and inoculation against dangerous diseases, they are still out there, and still very hazardous. Over the last twenty years our media, enamored as it is with a titillating story, has regaled us with horrific tales concerning the E.coli bacteria in our food supply, the tropical Ebola virus, the worldwide AIDS epidemic, and of course Lyme disease. Likewise, the recent revelations concerning the influence of the mercury preservatives present in many vaccinations, and their potential implication in the rise of some diseases, has focused increased attention on the issue of toxic exposure in our society. Each of these types of biological toxic influences, like heavy metals and chemicals, causes a stress response in the body.

The Trigger Factor: The Account Is Closed. The sixth factor is a trigger that sets this whole process in motion. It can be a single event within one factor (e.g., a car crash or other accident, acute illness, sudden toxic exposure) or the accumulation of the effects of a number of these factors acting together. Regardless of which scenario causes the response, the trigger is literally the last ingredient that breaks the bank, and permits our body to descend into a catabolic stress response and, usually, exhaustion.

The vast majority of us deal with varying levels of one, several or all these factors at one time or another throughout our entire lives. When they occur in combination, at intense levels, and for an extended period, they eventually form the combination which drags us into the exhaustion phase of GAS. Each of these factors MUST be dealt with if we are to reverse the destructive processes and make our way back to good health.

In other words, we cannot simply rely upon addressing just one or two of these factors with an individual herb/nutrient, suite of nutrients or other therapy to '*get us through*.' That is the same as using a therapy as a drug, and simply masks the true underlying problem, setting us up for potentially more serious problems down the road.

One of my primary teachers in the area of bioenergetic assessments and remedies, Dr. Robert Cass, ND, put this situation into stark perspective for us during an early class he taught. Drawing on his 30 years of experience as a naturopathic physician, he told us that when he first started practice in the mid-1970s, he was able to recommend one or two remedies to his patients and usually address the underlying problem completely. Today, however, the level of stress, especially toxic stress, has increased so greatly that the average person cannot deal with the situation effectively absent multiple remedies to address the multiple metabolic challenges facing them.

The Exhaustion Phase: We Declare Bankruptcy. When the body enters the "*exhaustion/fatigue phase;*" the combination of the types, intensity, and duration of the stress has overwhelmed the body's ability to cope. It is now unable to keep up with stress demands.

The adrenal glands, just like an exhausted sprinter, will run slower and slower, producing less and less of the adrenal hormones, and the glands themselves will start shrinking back from their enlarged state during the resistance phase toward their original size. This is also the phase where, because of the adrenal gland's exhaustion, the 'front office' of the hypothalamus and pituitary will be able to exert less and less control over them. It stands to reason; if the gland can't produce enough of its own hormones, it won't matter how much of the signaling hormones are produced by the 'front office.' Eventually, complete control will be lost.

The complete exhaustion of the adrenal glands, the point at which they completely stop functioning, is called "*Addison's Disease*" by the medical community. If the adrenal glands cease functioning and no action is taken, death will follow within a couple of weeks. Addison's Disease usually relegates a person to a life on a prescription of corticosteroid drugs, which over long-term use are extremely toxic to the liver, digestive tract, brain chemistry and eyes. Because they act as the equivalent of cortisol, they can also precipitate mood swings, depression and reproductive hormonal imbalances.

I had the unfortunate experience of seeing the effects of this type of treatment first hand. One of my close relatives, who suffered for many years from an autoimmune disorder brought on by adrenal exhaustion, had the misfortune of having to endure this treatment for over a decade. In the process, my relative experienced a myriad of symptoms, some physical, some emotional, which all but destroyed their quality of life.

But the effect of the exhaustion phase goes far beyond simply the adrenal glands themselves. Here's an overview of what typically happens to a person in the exhaustion phase of the stress response. If you think you're currently in the exhaustion phase of GAS, see how many of these characteristics apply to you.

Afternoon energy slump. Most likely, by about 2PM or so, they will be feeling its effects. That's because their adrenals now have reduced ability to produce adequate cortisol. Another term for cortisol is 'glucocorticoid,' because it is also integral to the proper processing of glucose, the primary energy producer in the body.

At the same time, their 'front office,' the hypothalamus and pituitary, are gradually becoming less and less capable of directing the adrenals to provide cortisol when they need it. Typically, I have seen the cortisol levels in a person with chronic adrenal fatigue reach their lowest levels around mid-afternoon. Even a flat-line cortisol profile will show at least some further dip in that time frame. The combination of their fluctuating blood sugar levels and the reduced ability of their 'front office' to help manage them leave them craving that afternoon pick-me-up of a cola and a candy bar.

Unfortunately, the caffeine and sugar combination only makes things worse, literally 'beating the dead horse' of their already exhausted adrenals. We'll talk about how to turn this situation around in a later chapter when we address needed diet and lifestyle changes. For now, keep in mind that *any* caffeine and/or processed sugar snack places demands on the adrenals in ways very similar to A'nath'a facing down that saber tooth.

Chronic fatigue not relieved by sleep, difficulty getting up in the morning, and weight gain. Because the typical sufferer of adrenal exhaustion has all but depleted their ability to manufacture needed cortisol in the right amounts at the right time, they are not able to enjoy a restful night's sleep. As a result, they literally crawl out of bed after a night of intermittent sleep, interrupted by continual awakening throughout the night. Once again, the body's chronic stress response is sabotaging their good health. While they deal with the stressors associated with their daily routine, their body's fight-or-flight response has mobilized their liver to provide a great deal of the body's glycogen reserves to convert into glucose and fuel their muscles to escape the 'threat.'

Unfortunately, the nature of the threat, usually in the form of the everyday stressors of their work routine, does not permit an actual physical escape. This has two significant and unfortunate consequences. First, when glucose is introduced into the bloodstream during the stress response, the body mobilizes the pancreas to secrete insulin to aid in the transport of the glucose into the cells. This is a simple description of how the body uses glucose in the blood to provide energy to itself. But in this case, the energy is not required (meaning the stress response will not be physically acted upon), so the cells do not easily accept the glucose. In response, the pancreas secretes even more insulin, attempting to increase the input to the cells.

A vicious cycle now ensues, which ultimately results in the oxidation ('rusting') of the cell membrane, causing even more resistance to the insulin. That's the actual name of this process: "*insulin resistance*," already identified by the health care community as a precursor to adult onset diabetes. The oxidation of that cell membrane also has detrimental consequences to the body's ability to maintain hormonal balance; more about that later.

But what happens to the glucose if it can't or won't be used by the body? We now have a situation where there is a large amount of glucose in the bloodstream with nowhere to go. Somehow the body must dispose of all this excess glucose. The body's innate self-regulating mechanism dictates that if it can't use a substance or eliminate it, the body must store it. Where does the body store excess glucose? In the fat cells!!! So the second consequence is unintended weight gain.

Thus we can clearly see the mechanism of how chronic stress is a major contributor to the epidemic of obesity in this country. The vicious cycle that is trapping people in adrenal exhaustion looks like this:

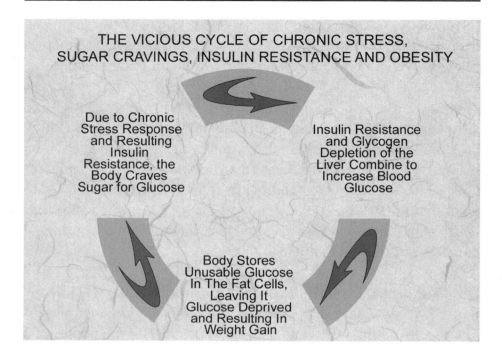

THE VICIOUS CYCLE OF CHRONIC STRESS,
SUGAR CRAVINGS, INSULIN RESISTANCE AND OBESITY

Due to Chronic
Stress Response
and Resulting
Insulin
Resistance, the
Body Craves
Sugar for Glucose

Insulin Resistance
and Glycogen
Depletion of the
Liver Combine to
Increase Blood
Glucose

Body Stores
Unusable Glucose
In The Fat Cells,
Leaving It
Glucose Deprived
and Resulting In
Weight Gain

It would not be as bad if the damage stopped there, but it doesn't. There is only a finite amount of glycogen (and, therefore, glucose) available in the liver at any given time. Absent a chronic stress response, the glycogen reserves in the liver are used during the sleep cycle to help repair and reconstitute the body. In fact, up to 60 per cent of the body's glycogen reserves are used during this repair and reconstitution phase at night.

But under conditions of chronic stress, the glycogen reserves in the liver become quickly depleted and are therefore unavailable during sleep. In its attempt to maintain balance, the body will nevertheless seek out these non-existent reserves during the night.

When the body discovers that the 'bank account' is empty, the adrenals will begin to secrete epinephrine in a vain attempt to help provide more glucose. This hormonal change is enough to wake people up, sometimes more than once a night. No wonder they're exhausted the next day! As a result of this process, they will routinely find themselves not fully awake until the middle of the morning (usually about ten AM).

Cravings for salt or salty foods. As the adrenal glands become progressively more exhausted, their ability to regulate the body's sodium levels diminish. That's because secretion of the adrenal hormone aldosterone, which regulates sodium and potassium levels, is also greatly diminished. This lack of sodium will be signaled by a craving for salt or salty foods.

Decreased productivity. This one should be a no-brainer for you. Since these people are already fatigued, they have limited energy to devote to the tasks that face them throughout the day. Most of us have experienced this feeling periodically; in the exhaustion phase of a chronic stress pattern the feeling is constant.

Decreased stress tolerance, increased effort required for daily tasks, lethargy (lack of energy), sweating easily. Typically, people in adrenal exhaustion tire very easily, finding it difficult to walk up even a couple of flights of stairs to their office. If they do, they finish breathing hard and sweating. Their capacity for additional physical work has been significantly diminished. People who sweat easily, and who find they have no energy reserves for daily tasks are very likely in adrenal exhaustion. Unfortunately, absent major intervention the situation is never relieved.

Dizziness/light-headedness when standing up quickly, swelling/ edema/water retention. An important part of the balance between sodium and potassium in the body is the ability of proper sodium levels to regulate blood pressure. When these sodium levels drop too low, as in a chronic stress response, the result can be a simultaneous lowering of blood pressure. The health care community calls this "*orthostatic hypotension.*" One of its most prevalent manifestations is dizziness or lightheadedness when standing up quickly.

At the same time, as the exhaustion phase continues to overtax the body, the 'front office' of the hypothalamus and pituitary will experience increasing difficulty controlling the proper secretion of aldosterone. The result can frequently be water retention.

Hair loss. This one may not be as easy to figure out. As mentioned earlier, the raw material which fuels the manufacture of adrenal hormones in the body is essential fatty acids (EFAs). A chronic stress response pattern consumes enormous amounts of these EFAs, much more than the average person takes in on a daily basis.

These same EFAs are also a valuable component of our hair. Remember again: the body will *always* fuel the fight-or-flight response first. So it stands to reason that if someone is not already consuming enough EFAs to fuel their stress response, their body will not provide enough EFAs to keep their hair healthy.

High blood pressure. This is definitely a result of long-term stress. Recall that when A'nath'a's stress response was activated, the hypothalamus not only caused the adrenal cortex to secrete the adrenal hormones cortisol, DHEA and aldosterone, it also caused the adrenal medulla to secrete epinephrine and norepinephrine.

If you watch any of the medical TV series, you know that the medical community uses epinephrine, also known as adrenaline, to help increase blood pressure in critically ill patients. In the presence of a chronic stress response, these hormones are in the bloodstream for longer and longer periods, ultimately driving up the blood pressure permanently.

High cholesterol, high triglycerides. Once again, look at the basic chemistry involving cholesterol and stress. Since cholesterol is the raw material for the stress response, and chronic stress generates a need for large amounts of cholesterol to make adrenal hormones, it makes perfect sense that the body will want to make more cholesterol. At the same time, if someone has been consuming high fat foods, which many stressed people eat for quick energy, the stress response will decrease the body's ability to clear the resulting triglycerides from their bloodstream.

High or low blood sugar. This one can be a little tricky, but it also makes perfect sense. When the stress response is initially activated, large amounts of glucose flow into the bloodstream. If someone stays in the resistance phase, where adequate cortisol was available, the blood sugar remains elevated for a while. However, as they regress toward the exhaustion phase, the body's ability to secrete adequate cortisol and, therefore, control the blood sugar deteriorates. The result: fluctuating blood sugar levels, depending on what the person ate and when. At this point, they are vulnerable to extreme swings in blood sugar, which are exacerbated if they happen to miss a meal.

Longer recovery time from illness, injury, or trauma. This is a logical outgrowth of the development of allergies and chemical sensitivities mentioned in the section on the resistance phase. If the attention of the immune system is primarily directed toward defending from external threats, it will be less able to mobilize its defenses to address illness, injury or trauma.

At the same time, the now low cortisol levels will have a very limited capability to combat pain and inflammation. Of the two, it is inflammation which is the more influential in affecting the length of recovery time. Remember: the fight-or-flight response always takes priority!

Poor circulation. Recall from Chapter 4 that the cardiovascular system transforms itself to provide increased blood supply to the muscles to allow the body to escape the threat; simultaneously, the blood vessels near the skin close down to prevent excessive bleeding from wounds. That means that other important functions get short shrift as well.

This is supposed to be a temporary situation. If allowed to continue over an extended period of time, this translates into systemic poor circulation, especially to the individual organ systems and the periphery of the body. Lack of adequate oxygen at the cellular level is implicated in the onset of a variety of serious illnesses, most especially cancer.

Bottom line: These people are in bad shape and getting worse! Let's take a look at their body, from top to bottom, system by system, as they go about their day:

- Their brain is operating as if they are fleeing a threat, all the time; they now have limited access to those parts of the brain that control the higher functions such as judgment, creativity and decision making. As a result, their thinking is becoming increasingly fuzzy.
- They are chronically depressed, and 'snap' at their co-workers. Kept up long enough, it may lead to the use of maladaptive coping strategies, such as passive-aggressive personality disorder, dissociative identity disorder, or post-traumatic stress disorder.
- Their eyesight is starting to deteriorate; they may need glasses.
- Their heart and lungs operate as if they are ready to flee, all the time, but their gradually increasing exhaustion makes them less and less capable of physical exertion. Their internal blood sugar management via the liver and pancreas are becoming less and less effective. Their cholesterol and triglycerides are elevated all the time.
- Their digestion and elimination are severely compromised. They are constipated nearly all the time, and may have to rely on laxatives.

- Their muscles and joints *ache!*

Obviously, these people need help. Unfortunately, on a daily basis they are typically walking into an environment, the offices of Corporate America, which offer little or no meaningful ability to permanently address these health challenges. In fact, as clearly demonstrated in Chapter 3, there is a very good possibility that the circumstances of their employment situation will contribute greatly to the worsening of their health situation, creating a health-related 'perfect storm.'

Many people start drinking alcohol to excess as a means of coping. They get depressed, find it difficult to sleep, experience chest pain. The body runs out of the immunity to fight diseases. What happens is that the body loses all its resistance in its effort to ward off the stress. Thus, very often, those under severe, prolonged stress may contract diseases related to immune deficiency and may even die of these diseases. Long-term stress can also be a contributing factor in heart disease, high blood pressure, or stroke.

So, very often, these persons die of diseases such as cancer, pneumonia, etc. For example, the Japanese phenomenon of *karoshi*, or death from overwork, is believed to be due to heart attack and stroke. For most people, though, the stress will never be identified as the cause of the death. Many researchers call stress the proxy killer. Some other disease always takes the blame for it.

But where does all this actually start? How do men and women each come to the point where stress has taken over virtually every activity of their waking (and sleeping) lives? As you might well expect, there are some significant differences between how men and women handle stress, and how it handles them. Turn the page to find out why this is so.

CHAPTER 6

STRESS AND GENDER:
HEAD IN THE SAND VS. CLIMBING THE SAND DUNE

"One gender is not better than the other. We are equal even as we are different; advantaged in some ways, at a disadvantage in others. And it's not as though we live in different realities. We see the same world. We just, on average, tend to focus on different parts of it. Accepting this helps us to cease trying to make each other more like ourselves."

— Paul and Sandy Coughlin, Married But Not Engaged

From the outset, we need to recognize that stress has significantly different physiological and hormonal effects on males and on females. That does not imply that chronic stress is any less detrimental to one or the other, however. As we shall see in this chapter, the differences arise as a function of the respective genders' hormonal systems and gender-specific life experiences. These factors, in turn, have a direct impact upon the level of chronic stress each person experiences, and determine what effect that stress level has on each person's state of health.

Why It Matters to America. As of October 2006, the US Bureau of Labor Statistics reported a non-farm workforce of 136,745,000 total workers, of which 65,945,000, or 48.2 per cent, were women. Since World War II, this number has been rising as women have continued to join the workforce, so that now men and women are contributing, almost equally in number, to the productivity of the American economy. As such, it is of crucial importance that organizational managers and leaders have at least a rudimentary knowledge of the essentially different effects of stress on the men and women in their companies, so they can more clearly comprehend where their health care dollars are being spent and why. This same body of knowledge is valuable to individuals as well. By better understanding the differences in how each gender reacts and adapts to stress, we can all better address the challenges those differences present. Before we can do that, though, we need to recognize and understand how stress can negatively affect each gender beginning in early childhood, thereby establishing lifelong negative physiological patterns.

Stress And Childhood: The Foundation Is Laid.   The foundation for hormonal disruptions can be established in the earliest phases of childhood. Applying the Stress Stack model, we can see that if these factors are of sufficient magnitude and duration, or overlaid with some sort of traumatic event, they can create a situation in the young child which easily overwhelms his or her growing body's ability to handle stress. Since every aspect of the child's brain and body are undergoing rapid change and development, it's important to understand and accept that children do not have the same ability as adults to understand what stress does to them, nor do they have the same ability to cope with stress. Some telltale signs that children are having difficulty dealing with stress are mood swings, night terrors, depression, decreased emotional margin and accompanying fatigue (usually represented by either an inordinate amount of required sleep to function or great difficulty awakening and arising in the morning). Additionally, the early formation of a chronic stress response, and the accompanying changes in the brain chemistry, will predispose the child to the various types of attention deficit disorders.

One all-too-common scenario that can result in a chronic stress response is living with ongoing physical, mental or emotional abuse at home, whether the abuse is directed at the child or not. For these and a host of other reasons, if the child's cognitive filter is predisposed to creating a chronic stress response (i.e., the 'ruts in the road' are already forming), s/he will move deeper into hormonal distress and show a gradual increase of the manifestations mentioned above. In many instances, it is the unceasing whirlwind of school and extracurricular activities and the inflated performance expectations of parents that combine to create this situation.

Author and researcher Joseph Chilton Pearce, in his landmark book *The Biology of Transcendence*, offers some convincing evidence of the negative influence of chronic stress on a child's ability to fully develop. He identifies several crucial phases of brain development throughout childhood and adolescence that will be negatively impacted by the presence of chronic stress. In particular, the development of the brain's prefrontal cortex, the portion of the brain that governs judgment, creativity and decision making will be stunted by chronic stress. This information has huge implications for the child's physiological development, as well as for her/his ability to reach maximum potential as a contributing member of American society.

The good news is that there are some very positive and effective means available to both assess the extent of the problem and do something about them early, before lasting damage is done. The assessment modality of adrenal hormone salivary testing, also called the Adrenal Salivary Index (ASI), can be accurately used on children as young as the age of four. This can provide an accurate assessment of the degree of hormonal distress the child is experiencing, which in turn can help a parent and their health care practitioner design a protocol to effectively address the problem. This issue and the potential solutions that are available will be addressed in more detail in Chapter 8. In regards to gender, it is from puberty onward that the paths of hormonal complexity begin to significantly diverge. It is from this point that we will address the differences in the effects of stress on each gender.

Stress and Males: The 'Head in the Sand' Syndrome. The *"hypnosis of social conditioning"* that today apparently governs the relationship between males and stress is that males are generally impervious to stress. This attitude usually first manifests during the puberty phase of development, when the male is asked to participate in activities that are generally defined as 'masculine,' such as competitive sports and organizational leadership. The common element in all these activities is a demonstrated ability to operate successfully under stress, and this attitude of apparent invulnerability carries over well into the adult years. While it is definitely a major contributor to a male's success in contemporary American adult life, it also has a significant down side.

Men come to believe that they should be able to endure stress without complaints, so they frequently take a 'head in the sand' approach, ignoring any problems that may arise such as adrenal fatigue, diabetes or cancer. The result throughout society has been the increasing prevalence of 'male menopause' or 'andropause,' evidenced by the huge market and media exposure for pharmaceutical drugs related to male erectile dysfunction (ED). Much of this condition is brought on by the *"pregnenolone steal"* that we discussed in Chapter 4, which accompanies any chronic stress response pattern.

Largely as a result of the attitude above, a number of experts now agree that male endocrine disorders are among the most under reported and misdiagnosed functional disorders in our society today. However, though the effects of stress are relevant to men, for two reasons we will only briefly address them here. First, men are generally much more hesitant to discuss the physical, mental and emotional manifestations of a chronic stress response (especially as it applies to sexual performance and response) with their health care providers than women are. As a result, we don't have as much data on this problem, so we can't discuss it in as much detail as we can similar problems that women experience.

Unfortunately, the predominantly male tendency to stoically endure such physiological disruptions not only denies them meaningful care, but precludes the ability to both accurately assess and address their health issues, thus setting them up for more serious health compromise as they continue to age. This is the most comprehensive explanation for why I have characterized males as having their 'head in the sand' when it comes to dealing with stress. It is also a major contributing factor to the increase in corporate health care costs. The fact that many males wait until the situation has become severe drives the cost of resolving the problem significantly higher.

This situation also occurs in large part from the phenomenon called 'creeping normalcy.' Most hormonal changes in the human body occur gradually, in many cases over a period of many years. As these changes occur, the innate wisdom of the body starts to make adjustments for the changes. These slow and subtle changes usually occur in small increments such that, combined with the hesitancy of men to report any problems, they cause little real concern. Since these changes typically occur against the backdrop of our contemporary society, with its built in set of 'normal' stress causing factors, there is a general acceptance of the inevitability of these physiological changes. For example, as a society, we have come to accept as a given that as men age, their ability to achieve an erection is progressively diminished. Ergo, the above-mentioned popularity of ED drugs. But is that truly 'normal,' or is it one more example of social conditioning? A look at some other cultures is very revealing.

Over the years, several researchers have traveled the globe and studied the longevity of aboriginal peoples. Their examinations of the Hunza people of northwest Pakistan were particularly revealing. Prior to the introduction of 'modern' Western food and health care, the Hunza men were routinely enjoying normal sexual relations well into their second century of life. Obviously, there was nothing 'normal' about ED in *that* society!

Second, the male endocrine system, in a physiological sense, is much simpler than the female. Therefore, it is much less prone to disruption from the stress-causing factors in the Stress Stack that we have talked about previously. This does not mean in any sense that males are immune from the ravages of chronic stress; far from it. It simply means that when a given stressor or set of stressors is equally applied to both male and female, the much greater complexity of the female endocrine system predisposes it to earlier and more noticeable disruptions than does the male. This is a physiological fact, not a social commentary.

The reason for this greater sensitivity, in contrast to the male, is that the female hormonal system displays much greater changes in hormone levels throughout a normal human lifetime. Because it is a much more dynamic system than the male, it presents many more opportunities for stress to negatively impact the woman. These disruptions can occur at virtually any point in a woman's life, but are more likely at points when significant hormonal changes are already taking place, such as puberty, pregnancy and menopause.

Therefore, the remainder of this chapter will be an adrenal hormone-related journey through the experiences of a typical woman's life. If you are a male reading these words, please do not mistake the description as being totally divorced from your experience. This chapter is valuable to you for two very important reasons. First, the effect on your hormonal balance varies from a woman's only in degree. While the physiological particulars are different, some of the major effects of chronic stress I will discuss are also relevant to you, and you therefore have much to learn from this chapter for yourself. Second, if you have a special woman or women in your life, the description of each phase can bring you a clearer understanding of their particular, age- and stress-related challenges and, therefore, provide you with powerful tools to more empathetically support them.

Stress: and Females: 'Climbing the Sand Dune'. The combination of stressors in our society has created health crises for millions of women that I liken to trying to climb a sand dune. With our societal overemphasis on quick fixes, we naturally gravitate toward those perceived health 'solutions' that are simple and quick. However, since most of them do not address the underlying foundational issues of a woman's health, they wind up creating situations where the woman feels better for a while, only to see her state of health slide slowly and frustratingly back to its previous compromised state, much like what occurs when a person tries to climb a sand dune, only to slide frustratingly back to where they began. If the foundational issues remain unaddressed for an extended period, the backward slide will accelerate, just like a fall from a sand dune, leaving women without the physical and emotional resources to successfully recuperate.

The Teen Years: The Damage Begins To Show. The situation for a young woman begins to complicate greatly when she enters puberty. Now, in addition to having to supply the increased load of adrenal hormones, her body is demanding a significant supply of pregnenolone to synthesize the testosterone, estrogen and progesterone needed for continued development and operation of her newly active reproductive system. This can easily overwhelm the body's ability to supply adequate raw material all at once, and frequently results in the new teenager enduring not only a chronic stress response, but difficult menses and fatigue throughout puberty.

A humorous but instructive story on this subject was related to me several years ago while I was flying as a first officer. The captain on that trip was bemoaning the fact that, once his daughter had reached puberty, she had become increasingly difficult to deal with.

He characterized it like this, *"Pete, the day my daughter had her first period was the day an alien being came to live in my house."'* The humorous aspects of this comment aside, is it any wonder that, with the stresses of contemporary life overlaying the important process of sexual development, any teenage girl would experience difficulty during this phase of her life?

A recent article in *USA Today* documented an even more graphic example of this phenomenon at work: the high number of female intercollegiate athletes suffering from depression. Can you 'connect the dots' with this one? Elite young female athletes, by their very nature overachievers, living in an environment characterized by constant time management challenges (school, sports and social life), greater-than-average daily stress on their bodies (via daily workouts, sleep deprivation, poor food choices and the other stress factors typical of college life), and a cognitive filter that is overwhelmed by the inputs presented to it. Result? Chronic *"pregnenolone steal,"* emotional problems, depression and fatigue. I have seen this regrettable situation more than once in my own practice. Two high achieving young women, both of whose cognitive filters were not well suited for dealing with the multiple stresses of university life, were wisely withdrawn by their parents temporarily from their respective universities so that their bodies could regroup from their overwhelming stress response.

Family and the Work Force: A Whole New Set of Challenges.
Once most women enter the work force, they are subjected to some of the same stress factors of the college coeds mentioned above, albeit from different directions. Combine the time management challenges associated with marriage/long-term relationships, family and workplace with a cognitive filter which demands 'perfection' in all these areas, and a foundation is laid for both early menstrual problems and later adrenal functional disorders. And yes, by menstrual problems I do mean PMS!

Think about it for a minute. If the body is already drawing most of its available pregnenolone to fuel the stress response, how likely is it that it will be able to provide adequate amounts of the right hormones, at the right time, to allow a normal menstrual cycle? This brings to mind the importance of the cognitive filter and Leon Chaitow's research into this area, which revealed one of the common factors in the emotional makeup of women suffering from autoimmune disorders is a very high desire for order, predictability and perfection. This predisposes them to exert a high level of effort to achieve those goals, thereby routinely overtaxing themselves and pushing their bodies down the road toward ill health.

The same can be said for women who are currently far from autoimmune distress, but are well down the pathway in that direction. The maternal instinct of "*sacrificing for my children*" has been enshrined in this society as a virtue, causing countless women to neglect their own health in headlong pursuit of "*a better life for my children.*" While the sentiment is noble, it is obvious that more emotion than logic is at work here. Although most mothers of this mindset believe they genuinely do have their children's best interests at heart, I invite them to stop, think, step back from the emotional involvement in this situation for a minute, and regain some perspective. Regardless of what you do for your children now, how grateful do you think they will be if, 10 or 15 years down the road, they have to push you around in a wheelchair because you've overtaxed your body such that you no longer can take care of yourself? Do you want them to bear that burden for the rest of their lives and yours? What kind of role model do you think that is for your children, i.e., *I am literally killing myself to show you I love you.* Do you want that to be your grandchildren's memory of you, if you last that long? Think about it!!!

An additional source of stress, surprisingly enough, has been the substantial removal of the '*glass ceiling*' for women in Corporate America. While undeniably providing them with heretofore unavailable professional opportunities, the downside is their subjection to all the same stressors endured by their male CEO counterparts. Again, because of their more complex endocrine systems, female corporate executives are likely candidates for increased exposure to stress related maladies, in relation to their male counterparts.

Women and Fitness: Too Much Of A Good Thing? The effects of stress on college athletes, described in a previous section, are also experienced long past a woman's teen years. For example, are you aware that many female long distance athletes, even those in their 30s and 40s, stop having their periods? If you guessed that this is due to "*pregnenolone steal,*" you were right on! And the reasons that occurs have implications not only for women's stress and reproductive health, but also for their cardiovascular health.

One of the most highly respected cardiovascular and aerobics research facilities in the country is the Cooper Aerobics Center in Dallas. They are uniquely equipped to conduct incredibly in-depth research on this topic, and they certainly have. A significant finding that has surfaced as a result of their research is that, after about 30 minutes of strenuous aerobic exercise, the body's fight-or-flight response kicks in, and the adrenals start to secrete their hormones in significant amounts. It is as if by running hard for those thirty minutes, suddenly our body's response shifted as if we were now lifting weights. Although you can continue to develop increased lung capacity by training longer than 30 minutes, the appearance of the fight-or-flight response means that there is accompanying inflammation, necessitating a rise in cortisol levels. This inflammation is systemic, negatively impacting cardiovascular health.

You may remember that, in the mid-80s to early 90s, there was a rash of deaths within the long distance running community, most notably the runner and famous author, Jim Fixx. The Cooper

Aerobics Center took it upon itself to solve this baffling mystery. After all, these people were generally considered to be among the healthiest and most fit on the planet. Why would they succumb to sudden death in this manner?

There were several theories offered, one of which was that Jim Fixx, having been a recovered smoker, was simply reaping the harvest of a formerly unhealthy lifestyle. The actual results surprised many. They showed that the cardiovascular systems of these people were more typical of the elderly than highly fit athletes. The reason? Their repeated, excessive long distance training predisposed their circulatory systems to inflammation, necessitating chronic activation of the body's fight-or-flight response. Once the inflammatory process started, the body's repair mechanisms kicked in, laying down irregular layers of fibrin (also known as scar tissue) in the cardiovascular system, which in turn became a convenient site for stray molecules of cholesterol and calcium to latch onto. This discovery has helped to change the health care community's understanding of the factors affecting cardiovascular disease, from the old congestive model to the new inflammation model.

Why did I bring up this subject? Because these same processes are active in women, especially female athletes. Another recent newspaper article detailed how an increasing number of accomplished, upper income women are turning to triathlons as both an enjoyable challenge and a way to remain fit. Given the information you've learned thus far, I'm sure you can see the risks here. Not only do they suffer an increased likelihood of developing cardiovascular disease, but the chronic activation of their bodies' fight-or-flight response also predisposes them to menstrual irregularities and, as we shall clearly see later in this chapter, opens the door to some serious potential health concerns as they age.

Stress and Pregnancy: The Hidden Hazard. Unfortunately, this unfolding process in a woman's body does not directly and physiologically affect just her. By that, I don't mean the emotional effect on her family and friends, although that is hardly insignificant! Nothing in her lifetime is more profoundly impacted by stress than a woman's pregnancy.

As I have mentioned earlier, I have been the beneficiary of many teachers as I have pursued my career in traditional naturopathy. One of the most influential has been Dr. I. Michael Borkin, Naturopathic Medical Doctor (NMD). Chairman of Sabre Laboratories, Director of The Foundation for The Advancement of Endocrine Research, and past President of the California State Naturopathic Medical Association, Dr. Borkin has been on the cutting edge of the effort to better understand the impact and interrelationships of the various endocrine organs on women's health. In the process, he has uncovered some significant information about the interrelationship of a mother and her developing fetus, especially as it pertains to the body's stress response.

In order to understand this process, we need to remind ourselves, at the most basic level, of the interrelationship between the woman and her developing fetus. The entire process of physiological change in a woman's body throughout her pregnancy is designed to provide a safe, nurturing, healthful environment for her developing child. That is why virtually every pregnant mother is advised to take good care of herself throughout the pregnancy: eat healthfully; get plenty of rest; don't smoke or drink, etc. These are all wise and helpful pieces of advice. But what about stress? This part of an expectant mom's lifestyle is virtually ignored. Yet, in my opinion, it has a more profound impact than any of the other factors on the likelihood of a successful delivery.

The reason is that an expectant mother under chronic stress significantly changes the experience and the outcome of a pregnancy, for both mother and child, in ways that most people are totally unaware of. As we discovered earlier, under stress, the body secretes a hormone called cortisol, which assists it in dealing with the pain and inflammation that accompanies the stress response, and helps optimize the body's use of glucose. When a body is experiencing chronic stress, conditions can be created which overwhelm the body's ability to secrete adequate cortisol. This is challenging enough for the average person, but can become almost insurmountable for the expectant mother.

How does this scenario unfold? A new mother under chronic stress will usually experience a very difficult first trimester, punctuated by frequent morning sickness, increased sensitivities to certain foods, and a general feeling of fatigue and unwellness. This is due to the fact that the developing fetus itself is adding a new source of stress to an already overwhelmed body.

As the pregnancy enters its second trimester, however, Mom starts to feel better. The placenta, the life-giving umbilical that connects mother and fetus, is now secreting about 450 milligrams of progesterone per day. Remember how I defined progesterone as a 'pinch-hit' hormone in Chapter 4? Well, during the second trimester it's at bat almost constantly in a stressed new Mom, being converted to cortisol to keep up with her stress demands. Keep in mind that the placenta is definitely a two way street. Although it is intended to help the mother provide the fetus appropriate sustenance, it also offers a pathway for the fetus to provide its mother what she needs, as well. The maternal body's fight-or-flight response is so powerful that it will even ask a developing fetus to help fuel it. In effect, the overstressed Mom is feeding off her developing child's hormones.

By the beginning of the third trimester, Mom is feeling *great!* The baby's fully developed adrenals are churning away to help Mom. In the process, however, the baby's adrenals actually *over*-develop, creating a condition the medical community calls *"hyperadrenalism."* Recall that this condition is normally found in the resistance phase of Hans Selye's General Adaptation Syndrome, discussed in Chapter 4. In other words, because Mom has been unable to effectively modulate her own stress response, she is bringing an already stressed-out infant into the world. It is a sad commentary on our nation that we are the only Western country which considers hyperadrenalism in newborn children a normal condition.

This unbalanced condition comes to a conclusion when the baby is delivered, with significant negative consequences for both mother and child. A newly delivered baby with overdeveloped adrenal glands is typically fussy, temperamental, and difficult for the new Mom to deal with, much like anyone who lives in the resistance phase of the stress response. That's because s/he is dealing with a set of adrenal glands of much greater size than her/his tiny body needs, and they are able to provide a *much* greater level of adrenal hormones than that little body is able to use properly. Manifestations of such a condition will include not only fussiness but, as the child grows older, emotional volatility inappropriate for its age. In other words, the "terrible twos" will come home to roost with a vengeance in a family whose young child is brought into the world in this way. Later on, this condition can also contribute to the manifestation of developmental problems, such as attention deficit disorder.

But the much bigger challenge is presented to the mother. At a time when her body is attempting to normalize itself hormonally, it is unable to do so. That's because the stress and reproductive hormones are derived from the same raw material, and the survival-related adrenal hormones will always be synthesized first. This condition was temporarily alleviated when the baby's adrenals were assisting

Mom, but now there is no help, and the already excessive stress level is greatly increased by the additional duties of new motherhood. Add to this the above mentioned temperamental newborn, and the stage is set for an all-too-common scenario: fatigue, mood swings, and episodes of depression, all manifestations of what the medical community calls post-partum depression. If there are other children in the home, especially younger children who demand greater attention, the stress load can become completely unmanageable. One young new mother I have dealt with called me in tears, asking for help in dealing with her overwhelming feelings of sadness. She was fearful of filling her medical doctor's antidepressant prescription because of the negative media revelations on its effects. But she also wanted something natural that would help her feel better *now*.

This heartbreaking situation brings up two important points. The first is that *prevention* is the best weapon we have to combat such a situation. If this young Mom had allowed me to work with her during her pregnancy to help better modulate her stress levels, she would have stood a much better chance of avoiding her postpartum health challenge to begin with. At the same time, her desire for immediate relief, while understandable, reflected a fundamental misunderstanding of how natural and alternative remedies actually work.

In so many respects, our society at its foundation has become a 'Fast-(fill-in-the-blank)' society.' By that I mean that we are not only a 'fast food' nation, but 'fast entertainment,' 'fast shopping,' we can just fill in the blank after 'fast.' In Chapter 2, I pointed out that our nation literally prides itself on being able to do everything fast; it is a primary measure of efficiency. That also includes health care. One of the time tested marketing ploys Big Pharma has always used is *"fast relief."* They have conditioned us (one more 'hypnosis') to believe that fast is *always* better. Many medical doctors will unhesitatingly agree with that statement. However, this mentality ignores the fundamental way in which the human body operates.

Hormonal imbalances which lead to situations like our young Mom's above, as well as millions of other unbalanced conditions in millions of other women, take months or years to develop. As such, their balance will *not* be favorably resolved in a matter of a couple of weeks. Make no mistake; antidepressants simply do *not* favorably and permanently alter one's underlying hormonal imbalance except in a very limited sense. Without addressing those foundational health issues that directly affect the imbalance you are, in effect, putting a Band-Aid on the problem, one which over time will become less and less effective.

The Later Years: Perimenopause and Menopause. Unfortunately, the hormonally related challenges women experience do not end with their child bearing years. In fact, one of the most health-crucial phases of a woman's life occurs as she enters menopause. It is here that the combination of the state of her body's stress response, the cumulative effect of all the factors of her personal Stress Stack that contribute to it, and the state of her own cognitive filter can combine to either allow her to easily navigate into post menopause or wreak devastating havoc on her health and relegate her to a remaining life of steady physical decline.

In order to fully understand how this all fits together we must understand how a woman's hormonal system is supposed to operate during this time. After menopause, the source of reproductive hormones should be the adrenal glands. Specifically, under normal circumstances the hormone androstenedione (if that name sounds familiar, it is an anabolic steroid formerly used by many elite athletes) is secreted by the adrenals and is then conjugated into the various estrogens, testosterone and progesterone. In adequate amounts, this permits the woman to enjoy a relatively stable transition into menopause and post menopause.

However, if the adrenals are compromised by chronic and protracted stress, and the cognitive filter itself is predisposed to a chronic stress response pattern, the body will be unable to synthesize the appropriate levels of hormones. Our old friend the "*pregnenolone steal*" will be busily at work, robbing the adrenals themselves of the ability to produce all the hormones the body needs. The woman may be able to produce adequate adrenal hormones, but reproductive hormones will be shortchanged.

However, in a great many cases, the adrenals have already descended into the exhaustion phase and are even unable to produce enough adrenal hormones to keep up with the demand. These are the people who are constantly fatigued, reliant on sugar and caffeine to 'get through the day,' and at constant risk of opportunistic and chronic infections. These women are also the ones who experience the full brunt of menopausal symptoms, a signal from their bodies telling them that their adrenals are severely depleted. This is also significant because the adrenals are a key component of the body's immune function. Given that this piece of the immune system puzzle is so critically important, ignoring it actually sets the body up for significant immune compromise later down the road (as mentioned earlier).

The results are usually a difficult menopause and post-menopause, punctuated by the notorious hot flashes, night sweats and mood swings, as well as increased vulnerability to a host of acute and chronic illnesses. A growing body of research reveals that chronic adrenal stress correlates directly to the challenges experienced during menopause. The explanation above tells you why.

It is primarily the fear of breast and uterine cancer, combined with the desire for relief of menopausal symptoms that usually motivates women to seek help in the form of hormone replacement therapy (HRT). Many women do feel better with this type of treatment

. . . for a while. But there are also significant pitfalls with electing this type of treatment that are not widely known. It is important, therefore, to have detailed knowledge of all available options before committing to a course of action. A mistake could, quite literally, greatly shorten one's life.

A recent study from the Women's Health Initiative concerning synthetic and non-human HRT revealed some startling, negative impacts of this type of treatment. What exactly did the study say? Simply put, the use of a primary brand of pharmaceutically supplied hormone therapy containing estrogen and progestin was found to significantly elevate postmenopausal women's risk of breast cancer, heart attacks, and strokes. The fact that the scientists conducting the HRT study halted it due to the observed increase in ill health brought on by the treatment speaks volumes about the dangers of this therapy. Despite these revelations, and the sometimes sad and catastrophic consequences accompanying them, some health care providers still elect to use these dangerous substances. That boggles my mind.

However, an important point to note is that a decision regarding whether or not to use HRT should be an informed one, to be made jointly with your chosen health care provider. In order to do that, it is important to do some research yourself regarding the advantages and disadvantages of this type of therapy. There are numerous informational sources that will assist you in this quest, so please ensure that you take the time to investigate all aspects of this therapy before making a decision.

At the same time, whether or not you decide to avail yourself of some sort of HRT, it will still be crucial for you to normalize your stress response. Generally speaking, what do we mean by that? First, the body's hormonal state must be accurately assessed by salivary testing of both the adrenal and reproductive hormones. While the medical community prefers the use of serum testing for hormonal assessment, this method reports the hormonal levels that have been conjugated by the liver and attached to proteins in the blood. In contrast, salivary testing reports the hormonal levels in contact with the body's tissues at the time the sample is taken. It's like the difference between watching a video tape versus a live report on the nightly news.

Second, once the results have been assessed, a targeted stress management, diet, lifestyle and supplementation protocol can be established that will rebalance the body's systems. This allows the body's own governing mechanisms to take over. Emphasis is placed on the proper functioning of both the adrenals and the liver, both of which play key roles in obtaining and sustaining overall hormonal balance.

The challenge of using this approach by itself for most women is that *it takes time*, and usually does not offer immediate relief from uncomfortable symptoms. Unlike hormonal replacement, which can show almost instantaneous results, and offer fast relief, all natural approaches require the body to "*entrain*" itself to the nutrients being offered. "*Entrainment*" means that the body's innate wisdom must identify the nutrient, decide what to do with it, and then employ it properly. This process can take up to 90 days to occur. In our 'Fast-(fill-in-the-blank)' society, that can frequently be challenging, especially since the manifestations of menopausal hormone imbalance can be so uncomfortable.

Please keep clearly in mind, however: the hormonal imbalances in a menopausal woman's body have taken, in most cases, a half century or more to develop; unless you want merely superficial results, they will not resolve themselves overnight. Because hormonal imbalances can take years to develop, it is not unreasonable for them to take a few months to resolve. I will offer some specific advice on how to find the right kind of help to accomplish this important work in the book's final section.

Soy: A Hazardous 'Do-It-Yourself' Choice. Because of the huge and sometimes bewildering array of women's health products available on the open market, some women with an evolved sense of self-empowerment (truly, hooray for them!) decide that, regardless of the complexities involved, this can be a successful do-it-yourself project. While I know there are some (my own wife included) who have indeed succeeded in this endeavor, most women who embark on this difficult venture rarely enjoy the degree of success they are looking for.

A big part of the reason for this is that there is so much conflicting and downright misleading information that is available about the subject of hormone balancing. Go to the Internet and there are literally hundreds of studies, some well conducted and some not, which purport to prove the effectiveness of various herbs, vitamins and minerals in addressing this problem.

Many medical professionals who read this book will now sit back with a self-satisfied smile and variations of the thought "*I told you so!*" My response is: not so fast, doctor! In my opinion, our medical/pharmaceutical research system is so outdated that it currently presents one of the primary impediments to delivering quality healthcare to menopausal women, and virtually anyone else, in this country. The discussion in Chapter 1 about 'advocacy science' clearly presents the reason why.

In the case of the use of herbs and nutritionals for the alleviation of menopausal symptoms, although there is much good information available about the effectiveness of such herbs as black cohosh and wild yam, no nutrient passes muster with the medical establishment because the research is not "*evidence based.*" No matter that many of these same remedies have been used with documented therapeutic results by billions of women around the world for, in some cases, *thousands* of years. Our self-appointed scientific superiority allegedly trumps all of that. Go figure. Because of the above, since most of us have little experience in evaluating the accuracy of published research, and since so much of that research is now tainted by financial influences, it is very difficult to judge which research is offering the most reliable information. This is especially true in the case of soy.

As the proponents of soy contend, it is true that soy has been used for thousands of years in Asian countries . . . as a condiment, in small quantities, and in fermented form, such as tempeh, natto, miso, soy sauce and (later) tofu. Nowhere throughout Asia do you see regular, widespread consumption of unfermented soy or soy products as a main portion of a meal. Additionally, the type of soy used in Asia is a completely natural form. Not so in this country. Many big agricultural/chemical companies in this country have jumped on the soy bandwagon, promoting it as a 'health' food. Adhering to the usual American consumer paradigm of *"more is better,"* the soy growers have convinced the FDA that a form of soy called GMO (for *"genetically modified organism"*) is safe for human consumption. A closer look at GMO soy tells a different story.

GMO soy is created by combining the genetic material of natural soy with that of some other plant or creature, usually to permit the growing soy plant to avoid such hazards as insect pest or bacterial infestations, or to enhance the inherent characteristics of the plant itself. Those are certainly worthwhile goals. However, it is the unintended consequences of these endeavors that create health problems for us all. Understanding this situation requires us to have some fundamental knowledge about the body's immune system.

At its most basic level of operation, the immune system works on the principle of finding, attacking and eliminating anything it identifies as 'other.' By that I mean that any substance that the body senses is foreign will activate an immune system response. Now, you tell me: can a plant created by splicing the genes of two or more living organisms be considered natural, or does it qualify as 'other?' Unfortunately, the body chooses the latter, and that is the primary disadvantage of GMO soy. It helps precipitate an unintended immune system response in the body.

But the bad news about soy doesn't stop there. Regardless of whether it's natural or GMO, one of the reasons why many women use soy products to attempt to balance their hormones is that soy is portrayed as being useful in that regard. And it's true: soy is considered a hormonal adaptogen, otherwise known as a selective estrogen receptor modulator (SERM). Two substances in soy, genestein and daidzein, act to either bring down high estrogen levels or raise low ones. However, the modulating effects of these two substances do not end when a woman's hormones reach optimal levels. If she continues to consume soy in significant quantities, she will take her hormones on a roller coaster ride. Additionally, because of the potency of these substances, they can also detrimentally impact the operation of the thyroid gland. As such, while I do use products containing soy in my practice, I do so for very specific reasons, in very limited quantities, and in very specific time frames.

There are several other reasons why regular soy consumption is not good for you. Studies have shown that soy increases the body's need for vitamin D. We are supposed to get the conversion of vitamin D we need from sunshine. Given the propensity of many people to remain indoors for extended periods, and the media-created hysteria over skin cancer, most women in this country already do not get adequate vitamin D. This is detrimental not only because it can be a contributing factor to mood disorders, but lack of vitamin D also contributes to poor calcium absorption, a major factor in the development of osteoporosis. Equally important, recent research has indicated that low vitamin D levels are implicated in the onset of both seasonal illnesses like the flu, and more serious diseases like certain forms of cancer.

Many people, especially vegetarians, consume soy for its protein and vitamin B12 content. However, they unfortunately do not realize that the form of vitamin B12 in soy is not absorbed by the human body and actually increases the body's need for vitamin B12. Given that vegetarians are at higher than normal risk for vitamin B12 deficiency, consumption of soy by them actually makes their situation worse.

When the interaction of soy with the human body was further examined, more negative effects were revealed. A study recently conducted at Brigham Young University revealed that animals fed with soy products showed elevated estrogen levels in the brain and a decrease in calcium-protein binding, negatively impacting brain function. Another study showed that soy interferes with protein digestion. In an important year long study conducted recently by the Israeli Health Ministry, researchers found *no* positive connection between soy consumption and relief of menopausal symptoms.

Unfortunately, it is almost impossible to get away from soy and soy byproducts in our food and personal use items. Look at virtually any 'health' food protein or snack bar on the grocery shelves and you'll see soy listed as a primary ingredient. The same can be said for a huge number of hair and skin care products. My wife and I searched for years to find a snack bar we could recommend to our clients that didn't include large amounts of soy.

As you can see by now, no matter how intelligent and well read you are it is very challenging to attempt to address the issue of hormonal health by oneself. This is especially true if someone is already in hormonal distress. The very things you try may wind up actually making the situation worse, not better. However, this does *not* mean that one shouldn't do their own research, ask questions, or try things they think may help them. The clients I most enjoy working with are those who are actively engaged in the process, ask penetrating questions, and read extensively about their health challenge. It does mean that one should seek out a qualified alternative health professional who can assist them with designing a program that fits their needs.

Autoimmune Disorders and Women: The Perfect Storm Becomes a "Coffin Corner." In aviation, there is a term used to describe very high altitude, slow speed flight that's called the "*coffin corner*." It's called that because if an aircraft is allowed to fly into that regime, it reaches a point where, if it tries to go higher, it will stall; if it tries to go lower, it will over speed. Either way, it will fall out of the sky. Health wise, the menopausal and postmenopausal phases of life can potentially be a woman's "*coffin corner*." If she has consistently overstressed her body over the years, for whatever reasons, the resulting stress and reproductive hormonal deficits, accompanied by a compromised immune system, can open the door to the onset of a variety of serious health disorders and leave the woman with no meaningful bodily reserves to fight against them. Said another way, menopause is the point in a woman's life where she can either step briskly into middle age, or paint herself into a literal "*coffin corner*" from which, ultimately, there is no escape.

This situation is most graphically illustrated in Chapter 3 by the dilemma that female flight attendants confront. The combination of the very stressful factors they contend with on a daily basis can and does create serious metabolic and hormonal imbalances which accelerate their progression toward the "*coffin corner*." I cannot begin to tell you the number of flight attendants I have encountered who either currently suffer from, or have suffered from, some type of stress related ailment; in the medical community these are usually lumped into the category of "*autoimmune disorders*." The list reads like a textbook on the subject: cancer (yes, cancer is an autoimmune disorder!), chronic fatigue syndrome, fibromyalgia, lupus, mixed connective tissue disorder, multiple chemical sensitivities (MCS), multiple sclerosis (MS), scleroderma, and many more. And there are countless others I have encountered who simply 'don't feel good.'

The medical community spends a great deal of time sorting and sifting through the specific symptoms and signs that correlate to a given condition, all so they can put a *name* to that condition. When a medical doctor presents a diagnosis to a patient, it is usually with the words "*You have (fill in the blank)*."

Deepak Chopra MD has some powerful words of wisdom that address this subject:

"*Scientists have shown that mental events transform themselves into molecules. These molecules are literally messengers from inner space. They are the equivalent of thought. When they were first discovered, they were called neuropeptides because they were initially found in the brain. Now we know that these neuropeptides are not confined to the brain, but permeate every cell in the body. To think a thought is to practice not only brain chemistry, but body chemistry. Every thought you have, every idea you entertain, sends a chemical message to the core of cellular awareness.*"

Think for a moment how that applies to the situation in the doctor's office above. While it may be superficially gratifying to put a name to why we don't feel well, the *manner* in which that information is conveyed sends exactly the wrong message to help us overcome our health challenge. By taking in the doctor's message literally (e.g., "*I HAVE cancer*"), we are sending a message to the core of our being that this is a part of us, and actually *belongs* there. I get so frustrated when I hear people talk about their health challenges in possessive terms, e.g., "*my arthritis*." All they are doing is making it less likely that their bodies will eventually want to let go of this health challenge.

This concept has been enshrined in many drug commercials aired by pharmaceutical companies; as you might expect, they have no objection to continuing with the use of such imprecise and harmful language. It helps them sell more drugs. If there is one area where the conventional medical community needs to improve its training, it is in the area of using accurate and *positively enforcing* language when conveying information to their patients. There is a huge difference between "*You HAVE cancer*," and "*the medical diagnosis is cancer*." The personal connection, or lack thereof, could make all the difference in the eventual outcome. I'll step off my soapbox now, and get back to the subject at hand.

In contrast to the medical approach, the traditional naturopathic approach steps back from the individual 'trees' that are the medical signs and symptoms, and looks at the whole 'forest' that comprises the client's health. In the process, we can help the client determine what underlying factors are at work to create the health imbalance they are addressing. When working with any client with a medically diagnosed autoimmune disorder, I have found that six such important underlying factors will inevitably surface: *a compromised digestive and eliminative system; suboptimal liver function; exhausted adrenal glands; weakened immune system function; chronic inflammation; the presence of the 'trigger factor.'* Of course, each of these factors can arise independently of an autoimmune disorder, but most or all of them usually accompany an autoimmune disorder. Most of the clients I have seen with such problems are women.

Digestion and Elimination: Cracks in the Foundation. The first underlying factor is a compromised digestive and elimination tract, the two foundational elements of good health. Usually because of poor dietary choices over the years, encompassing all the 'usual suspects' (i.e., caffeine, artificial sweeteners, processed sugar, white flour, and trans fats), the ability of the digestive tract to effectively absorb nutrients has deteriorated. As a result of chronic stress, the interior of the small intestine, responsible for absorption of nutrients, will swell and distort. As a result, the nutrients, which are supposed to pass through specifically shaped holes in the track (much like the baby toys which teach children shape correlation) can no longer accurately fit into those now-distorted holes. In many instances, the ability of the small intestine to absorb can be compromised by as much as two thirds. In other words, you can only absorb about a third of what you eat.

At the same time, those same poor dietary choices create a predominantly acid condition which both taxes the body's ability to remain in a healthful alkaline state, and gradually wears away the mucosal lining of the gut track. Over time, the thinning of this mucus lining can create a condition called "*leaky gut*," which now allows partially digested food particles to enter the bloodstream. When they migrate into the body's cell structure and lodge there, the body senses them as 'other,' and marshals the immune system to remove them. Thus can begin the process of 'autoimmune' response, including an increased secretion of adrenal hormones.

Remember from Chapter 4 that one of the functions that the fight-or-flight response *temporarily* shuts down is elimination. By the time a person with a medically diagnosed autoimmune disorder walks through my door, they are usually chronically constipated from the constant activation of the fight-or-flight response. The body is expending so much energy escaping the threat that it has little left to take care of the demands of elimination.

The Overtaxed Liver: Too Heavy a Load. Because of the stress that poor diet has placed on it, the liver struggles to keep up with the ever-increasing demands of detoxification. Simultaneously, it is unable to handle both that load and the need to manage the increased level of adrenal hormones. As a result, the effectiveness of the processes of detoxification and hormonal conjugation both suffer. Therefore, the stage is set for both hormonally related complications and the beginnings of the effects of toxic saturation.

Most of my clients who struggle with these issues are so-called "*universal reactors*," women who suffer exaggerated responses to the introduction of even very small levels of detoxification therapies.

That's because the liver, already overloaded with toxic/hormonal material, almost literally shouts "*Whoopee!*" at the prospect of any measure of assistance. The body overreacts to the therapy, releasing toxic material in an amount disproportionate to the stimulus in an attempt to alleviate the accumulated toxic burden. This of course results in the woman feeling poorly.

People who are not adequately familiar with the operation of their own bodies can sometimes react with the assertion, "*the stuff you gave me made me sick!*" In reality, their reaction to the therapy is a clear indication of the high levels of toxic material their bodies are carrying, and the need for the practitioner to proceed very carefully so as not to overwhelm the body's ability to handle the toxic load. It is not unusual for someone like this to take several months to recondition their system so that the liver is able to function properly. They must start with very small amounts of the detoxifier and gradually work their way up to the recommended levels as their liver can handle the increased load. This must be successfully completed before they can proceed with any other therapies.

This brings up a very important point, one which is virtually lost and ignored in the contemporary medical community. As the human body peels away the various layers of toxic influences, much like peeling an onion, it almost literally travels back through time, revisiting the circumstances which resulted in the toxic infestations to begin with. It is not unusual for a client to experience a brief return of the manifestations of each of those infestations as a result. Dr. Bernard Jensen, DC, a pioneer in the field of detoxification, called these episodes "*healing crises*," steps along the path to better health that are indications of the body ridding itself of toxins.

The corollary to this phenomenon is the misconception most people hold of the path to good health as being a linear progression from illness to wellness. That misconception has been reinforced by the medical community's insistence on using treatments which suppress symptoms, resulting in the patient feeling better *now*, but burying the cause of the symptoms ever deeper in the body, only to resurface in a later, more damaging form. With few exceptions, properly administered detoxification therapies will result in one or more of these "*healing crises*." Those exceptions are certainly worth noting, and I'll discuss all of these therapies, and the differences in how they work, in the final section.

Exhausted Adrenals: Barely Running At Idle. In the aviation world, one of the most potentially dangerous events is if a jet engine is allowed to over speed. It can, if allowed to continue unaddressed, result in the destruction of the engine and, sometimes, the airplane itself. Once over sped, the engine needs repair before it can resume normal operation. It would have difficulty even operating at idle. With all autoimmune disorders, the adrenals operate much like that, having already moved into the exhaustion stage. They have literally over sped themselves and can no longer function adequately. Adequate quantities of neither cortisol, DHEA, aldosterone, epinephrine, nor any other adrenally secreted hormone are available. The body's ability to respond to stress is severely compromised.

The Overwhelmed Immune System: TOO Outward Directed. Recall from Chapter 4 that during the stress response the immune system's function becomes outward directed, operating most efficiently at the periphery of the body to protect against the effects of wounding. In the case of any autoimmune disorder, another component surfaces: the immune system is on hyper alert, almost spring loaded to attack virtually anything that looks like a threat.

Chronic Inflammation and Pain: A Natural Outcome. Remember that a primary function of the adrenal hormone cortisol is to combat pain and inflammation during the fight-or-flight response. If the adrenals are no longer able to provide cortisol in adequate amounts, it stands to reason that the body will begin to experience gradually increasing levels of inflammation and pain.

The Trigger Factor: The Catabolic Stress Stack Model in Action.
Whether it is a single traumatic event or a combination of stressors whose inputs have overwhelmed the body, the sixth common element for any autoimmune sufferer is the presence of some sort of trigger mechanism, literally the "*straw that broke the camel's back.*"

As I repeatedly stress throughout this book, I believe that one of the primary reasons the medical community has been so minimally successful in addressing this category of ill health is that they have persisted in taking a "*magic bullet*" approach, i.e., trying to find one drug or therapy that can do it all. As you can see, this scenario presents both client and practitioner with multiple challenges that must all be addressed. Unfortunately for both client and practitioner, by the time a woman typically seeks help for one of these complex disorders, she is already in such a depleted state of health that she perceives herself as neither physically nor emotionally capable of handling anything even remotely this complex. It takes all of the practitioner's strategizing, counseling and coaching skills to help her successfully overcome these challenges.

The female life experiences such as puberty, pregnancy and menopause, as well as the male experiences such as andropause and ED, present significant health challenges to every person experiencing them, some of which cannot be overcome solely by self-help measures. The good news is that there are helpful solutions that can effectively address every one of these challenges. In order for these solutions to work, some important factors in our daily lives must first change. Turn the page to learn how to identify what these important factors are and, of equal importance, how we can effectively deal with them on our way to meaningful change.

Part Three

Taking Back Control

CHAPTER 7

LAYING THE FOUNDATION:
ADDRESSING THE ISSUE OF CHANGE

"There is nobody who totally lacks the courage to change."

— Rollo May

Where We Go From Here. In this final section of the book, we will be building the foundation of a program, and its particulars, to address the pandemic of chronic stress that, as you have seen, afflicts our society on so many levels. To do so, in this chapter we will first tackle the issue of change, and the societal, institutional and individual challenges and obstacles facing us as we implement it on our way to an effective stress management program.

In Chapter 8, we will then discuss the importance and means of developing a sense of self-empowerment, both as an organizational manager and as an employee/consumer, to tackle the challenges presented by chronic stress. We'll also address the issue of cost, and answer the important question of whether preventive CAM care should be classified as an expense or an investment for both organizations and individuals. Then we'll lay out the detailed recommendations for implementing both a personal and organizational program of preventive stress management.

In Chapter 9, using what we have learned thus far as background, we will lay out the organizational and societal changes, in the form of a series of government policy recommendations, that need to be implemented to better combat the detrimental impact of chronic stress on our society as a whole, and provide you with the means of making your own voice heard on these important issues.

Putting It All In Context: Increase Your Awareness. Once you have digested the contents of this chapter, with all of the hindrances to change that exist at every level of society, it all may appear overwhelming, that there is too much for one person to change, so remaining in precontemplation mode (i.e., inaction) is the best answer. But please keep in mind that I am not offering this information to discourage or disempower you. Quite the contrary. It is being presented so you will be better able to navigate your way toward your goal: creation of your own effective stress management program. By being better aware of these obstacles, some well known, some not, you will be better able to know where you can find meaningful help, and where you may be wasting your time.

The Importance of a Comprehensive Approach. Having absorbed the information offered thus far, you're beginning to understand the folly and shortsightedness of the 'patch-'em-up and-get-'em-back-to-work' philosophy that underlies the medical/pharmaceutical/insurance complex in America today. On its surface, it may appear to be cost effective; however, the collective experience of thousands of American corporations, small businesses, other organizations, and consumers over many years says otherwise. Remember, the American Institute of Stress reported that stress related ailments cost companies over $300 billion a year in increased absenteeism, tardiness, reduced productivity, and the loss of talented workers. Many of those lost workers, having succumbed to the "*Trigger Factor*" and descended into chronic illness, become part of the population that, according to a study by Harvard University, experiences the leading cause of financial bankruptcy in the US: inability to pay their medical bills. Have we seen any information that indicates a substantive change to that situation? I think you'll agree, the answer is a resounding *no*.

What does that translate into on a daily basis? We've seen earlier that over a million US workers a *day* miss work from health concerns whose root cause is stress. How many expensive employee visits to doctors and hospitals has that resulted in with no meaningful resolution of these employees' health concerns? According to the *2010 National Health Interview Survey*, conducted by the Centers for Disease Control, American adults paid over 229 million visits to doctors during the last year. Applying Miller's and Smith's estimates from Chapter 2 of what percentage of those visits were stress-related yields a figure of between 172 million and 206 million being caused by stress.

Likewise, how many prescription drugs have been dispensed to treat symptoms of chronic stress, with no meaningful impact? While cost figures are not readily available, the *2008 National Ambulatory Medical Care Survey* disclosed that 2.3 billion drugs were ordered or provided as the result of a doctor's visit, and an additional 280 million were provided via hospital visits during that year. In each case, three quarters of the visits resulted in the administration of drug therapy. Again applying Miller's and Smith's estimates, that means that approximately 1.72 billion to 2.1 billion drugs were dispensed to treat stress related complaints during visits to physicians, and 210 million to 252 million drugs were dispensed by hospitals for similar complaints.

If you are an organizational leader or manager, how many valuable employees or workers have *you* and your organization lost because of chronic stress? And how much of the cost of the treatments above were absorbed by *your* company?

This situation clearly demonstrates a stark and uncomfortable truth: neither conventional medicine, nor the natural health world, offers a means to simply prescribe our way to good health when dealing with chronic stress. Again, there are no 'magic bullet' products or therapies which can quickly, simultaneously and effectively address *all* the stress-causing factors in the Stress Stack we have previously uncovered. We must comprehensively and individually address all of them over time if we are to obtain workable solutions to this complex problem. In order to do that, we must also identify and address the societal and individual obstacles to successful implementation we will encounter along the way, and devise practical strategies to recognize and overcome or avoid those obstacles. Only then can we embark on a path that fits our organizational culture, makes sense to us personally, and is applicable and effective in our environment.

In other words, a holistically structured health *maintenance and prevention* program must take into account *all* the factors I have introduced in the Stress Stack model, include comprehensive solutions for each of them which will work in today's societal and business environment, and take into account the counter-conditioning factors that may stand in the way of our success. Because stress is a holistic phenomenon, it does not lend itself to effective alleviation by addressing only one or two factors. As evidence of the accuracy of that statement, I offer the year-over-year persistence of the factors that the APA identifies annually as causes of stress, most with no meaningful amelioration or alleviation from year to year. It's obvious, therefore, that we can't take a 'fast food' approach to the phenomenon that is chronic stress and expect to be successful.

It is also critically important at this juncture to realize that the recommendations offered in the chapters of this section are guidelines for constructing a program for *recovering from or preventing* the effects of chronic stress. They are *not* offered as a means of *withstanding* the effects of existing chronic stress in our society, much of which is physiologically and psychologically unendurable over time. You'll recall that Chapter 5 was devoted in its entirety to an in depth discussion of the effects of the exhaustion phase of the stress response. It provides compelling evidence that our societal stress load is, indeed, unendurable over the long term.

As we move forward with our discussion, the key lesson for organizational managers to absorb is that the current methods which their workers use to cope with stress are ineffective and largely broken. If they were not, the American workforce would not be hemorrhaging jobs overseas, and the American business community would not be continually and futilely engaged in the vicious cycle of demanding ever increasing productivity from a continually shrinking and chronically overstressed workforce.

At the same time, the key lesson here for individuals is that our bodies, and that of our families, friends, neighbors and coworkers, have clearly definable and finite limits which, if we breach them, mark the starting point of a cascade of health problems. The inevitable culmination of this cascade is serious illness and greatly increased health care costs that directly and negatively impact both our own personal, and our organization's, bottom line.

Since we are presenting information that impacts both organizations and individuals, we will take a dual track approach, addressing the larger, organizational context of each facet first, and then the individual context. It is important that we understand both, since the effects of stress on each member of our society exert a direct impact both on the ability of the organization to which the member belongs to accomplish its objectives and, in a very direct sense, on its bottom line. At the same time, the discussion provides organizational managers an opportunity to educate themselves about how both organizations and individuals respond to these situations, and what can be done to implement meaningful change in these areas.

The Strong Foundation: Not What You Might Think! In the American business community, an entire industry, management consulting, has grown up around the need for corporations to become more nimble, agile, and flexible in the rapidly changing business environment they inhabit. The management consultants who offer solutions to corporate business challenges effectively address virtually every aspect of their clients' operations and organizational structure save one: the health care benefits they provide to their employees. Yet this is the very area which generates the most profound change throughout an organization, and over which corporate managers perceive themselves to have the least control. That perception is an illusion, fostered by the managers' own lack of knowledge of other alternatives, and perpetuated by the providers of the benefits themselves: the medical/pharmaceutical/insurance complex. As we have seen, the tools that the medical community employs to deal with chronic stress are limited. As we shall see in this chapter, there are compelling and disturbing reasons for that which have huge implications for our collective future, and which we must take into account as we build our stress management program.

Despite what they might think, corporate managers *do* have the capability to effect change in this area, and that change begins the creation of a strong foundation of cost-effectiveness for the company and better health for its employees. In order to successfully effect that change, organizational managers must display a *significant desire for change* in the area of health benefits, the *willingness to empower the organization* with new knowledge and skills so that the change can have the desired effect, and the subsequent *willingness to invest the company's financial resources* in a program that has a high probability of achieving the desired results.

As we will see throughout this discussion, the same principles that govern the implementation of a successful organizational stress management strategy are the ones that determine success on an individual level. Therefore, on an individual basis, I repeatedly emphasize to my clients that building a workable stress management program always begins with building a strong foundation. Like building a house, one cannot devise a workable strategy for better health in any respect based solely on quick and easy fixes. Despite the declarations of some of my colleagues within and outside the natural health field to the contrary, the foundation for recovering one's health from the effects of chronic stress exists neither in the colon, nor the liver, nor even the adrenals. It can be found, first and foremost, in the mind of the person seeking help.

The most essential elements that contribute to a workable individual stress management program are a *significant desire for change* in one's state of health, the *willingness to empower oneself* so that the change can have the desired effect, and the subsequent *willingness to invest one's personal effort, energy and financial resources* in a program that has a high probability of achieving the desired results. I have discovered from extensive professional and personal experience that any client who begins a health improvement program with a firm commitment to these principles will enjoy a very high probability of success.

Conversely, if any of these three elements are missing, in either an organizational or individual context, the likelihood of success is very low. Let's take an in depth look at how these principles interface with the reality that confronts our society, and those organizations and individuals that inhabit it.

The Process of Change. Any program to improve organizational efficiency or individual health, regardless of its degree of complexity, involves behavioral change. Whether we are implementing new management policies, taking a prescription drug, changing our diet, or getting more exercise, the fundamental similarity among these activities is that we are being asked to change our behavior. On the surface, this appears to be a relatively straightforward process. We are essentially being asked to learn and apply new information and/ or newly acquired tools to our betterment. But is it really that easy?

Perhaps the most comprehensive explanation of the details of this change process in a health care context has been offered by Professors James O. Prochaska, PhD. & Carlo C. DiClemente,

PhD. Called the "*Transtheoretical Model*," it was derived in the late 1970s and early 1980s as a way to explain the process which governs any change in our behavior. As such, it offers us both a road map to the change process, i.e., a means to gage the likelihood of our own success if we undertook change in our current mental and emotional state, and a road map to changing our mindset so that any anticipated change we undertake has the maximum probability of success. Over time, this model has been demonstrated to have applicability to a variety of situations, within the health care system and outside of it, and at both organizational and individual levels.

Prochaska and DiClemente identified five discrete thought process phases we pass through on our way to meaningful change: *precontemplation; contemplation; preparation; action; and maintenance.* The first, *precontemplation*, is essentially maintenance of the status quo. As applied to organizational management of employee chronic stress, it is the stage where managers either don't recognize there's a problem with the stress levels of their employees, believe that the stress level experienced by their employees is manageable and not harmful, or believe that the currently available coping strategies are adequate for all their employees to deal with their current level of stress. A prevalent manifestation of organizational precontemplation is institutional inertia, characterized by the mindset of "*that's the way we've always done things here!*" The practical result of all these beliefs is that nothing is changed. Examples of organizational precontemplation abound throughout our country. In my opinion, any organization that responds to the continual rise in health care costs by spiraling ever more rapidly into the vicious cycle described in Chapter 2 is deeply mired in precontemplation mode.

As applied to dealing with the individual effects of chronic stress, it is the stage where employees either don't recognize that there is a problem with stress, believe that their level of stress is manageable and not harmful, believe that their current coping mechanisms are adequate to deal with their current level of stress, or simply have given up, believing that their situation does not lend itself to a solution. Other descriptions of the latter can include *"learned helplessness"* (i.e., *"It's not my fault, and I can't do anything about it"*) or *"inertia"* (*"It's just too hard and/or expensive to make changes!"*).

A prime individual example of precontemplation sat across the aisle from me on an airline flight a while back. Well dressed and groomed, the gentleman nevertheless tended to speak in a very loud tone of voice. Sitting on his seat back tray table, next to his laptop computer, was a huge personal coffee cup, the equivalent of three to four normal cups, which he obviously takes with him on business trips. As the flight attendant came by to take his drink order, he pointed to the cup and said loudly *"Just keep it filled. I have a lot of work to do!"* He obviously believed that his selected strategy of dealing with stress, over consumption of caffeinated beverages, fulfilled his needs. Recall from Chapters 1 and 3 my description of the effects of caffeine on the body; I have often wondered in what state his health is today.

The second phase, contemplation, includes those organizations and individuals who are thinking about change, but may be somewhat ambivalent about it. From an organizational management standpoint, this includes, for example, benefits program managers or human resource directors who want to address the problem, but feel either too ill-informed, overwhelmed by the task, or disempowered to do anything meaningful about it.

Many of these organizations and individuals are constantly seeking more information about a problem, but nothing ever seems enough. In business management terms, they are seeking what's called *"perfect information,"* an assurance that whatever solution they choose is absolutely guaranteed to be the right one. Understanding the intersection of the complexities of health care management *and* stress management can be so daunting that the average corporate benefits employee may make the internal decision to just 'go with the flow,' take what the marketplace will offer and not demand more. Additionally, senior organizational managers (i.e., CEOs or presidents), with their eyes forever focused on the bottom line, and using the same "*hypnosis of social conditioning*" regarding health care as their benefits employees, may demand an unattainable, virtually perfect standard of evidence that new, alternative therapies outside the medical model work before they will agree to incorporate them into their health care benefits programs. In the area of stress management, using those criteria, and that knowledge base, is a lot like going to the hardware store to buy oranges.

However, any well informed business manager will tell you that there is always a cost for obtaining perfect information; it is usually paid for in an increase in the costs of implementing a decision, or in the loss of the opportunity altogether (e.g., a competitor beats us to the market with a rival product). In a corporate benefits context, it usually results in the situation we see with the current corporate health care management system, i.e., ever rising costs and no meaningful change in the system. What we are really talking about here is risk management, and the primary drivers of the assessment of risk in these situations are the levels of knowledge of the people making those decisions.

From an individual standpoint, it can also include individuals who recognize they have a problem but, again, feel too ill-informed, overwhelmed or disempowered to address it. The cost can be procrastination to the point where major health challenges arise that could have been dealt with much more easily at an earlier point in time. I have seen quite a few prospective clients sabotage themselves in this way; they usually end a conversation about making substantive, positive changes to improve their health with "*I'll think about it.*" Again, the ability of the individual to move forward from this phase depends upon their level of knowledge, degree of "*hypnosis of social conditioning*" with respect to the medical/pharmaceutical/insurance complex, and tolerance for risk in this area.

Preparation is the third phase of the change process. During this time, a firm decision on a direction of movement has been made, and plans have been formulated. Organizational managers in this phase may have had the good fortune to obtain reliable information on effective stress management strategies, and are actively paring down the options to come up with a workable plan. Individuals may have identified a practitioner and formulated a preliminary plan of action ("*I'm going to call that naturopath and make an appointment tomorrow!*"). These are the people who may have already tried other health improvement strategies before, but were not successful in addressing the problem.

However, it is very easy for either organizations or individuals to fall into an insidious mental trap. A manager who has been culturally conditioned by the medical/pharmaceutical/insurance complex to expect the same level of performance from alternative therapies as they have come to expect from prescription drugs may set unrealistically high performance expectations for proposed changes, or expect too much progress in too little time from those therapies. If they are not willing to give new programs the time necessary to demonstrate effectiveness, they will pull the plug prematurely, and the failure of the new program will become a self-fulfilling prophecy. Organizational managers must judge the success or failure of new programs through use of realistic evaluation parameters having to do directly with the programs themselves, and not allow other factors (e.g., previous experience with the medical system or quarterly financial performance) which are not germane to the evaluation process to drive results.

On an individual basis, especially if people have been struggling with their situations for a long period of time, their emotional state primarily reflects both the frustration that they have been unable to successfully address the problem, and frequently a diffuse anger (at themselves, at health care practitioners who have previously been unsuccessful at helping them, at the 'unfairness' of the situation, etc.) which can cloud their judgment. This is usually reflected in self-talk or overt statements such as *"I'll give this program 30 (or 60, or 90) days. If it's not working by then, it's not working."*

Never mind that it's taken them their entire lives to reach this state of health, or that their time frame is totally arbitrary (i.e., based not on knowledge of the facts, but rather on individual preference, an emotional reaction, or personal convenience). It sets them up for further frustration and failure, and a return to either the contemplation or precontemplation phases, usually with the attitude of *"Nothing's going to work, so I may as well just give up,"* another manifestation of learned helplessness.

This brings up an important point about the change process that applies to both organizations and individuals: it is very easy for both to move forward *and* backward along the scale of the change process. They may reach a point where their cognitive filters either collectively or individually create the perception that there isn't a clear path to success available. To avoid this pitfall, they must be both very clear about their goals and motivation, and be willing to make the effort to adequately inform themselves about the situation in order to make wise decisions.

The fourth phase of the change process is *action*. This is where we actually put the plan into effect and begin making overt changes in our behavior. At this point, resolving the problem becomes the main focus of our attention and effort. In an organizational context, this is where benefits managers will have already constructed the program and are now explaining it and implementing it with both senior management and their fellow employees. At this point, it is extremely important to remember that this change process applies to all employees, and that each individual in the organization is at their own unique point on the change spectrum. Therefore, to create large scale compliance with the program the organization must account for employees in every phase of the change process in order for its program to be effective.

In an individual context, this is where your new program's rubber meets the road. The watchwords here are enthusiasm, consistency and patience. The tools we will use are those we will learn about in the next chapter. The goal is to make what you do a habitual part of your lifestyle, not just something you do occasionally. A senior executive from a natural products company I'm familiar with has some wise words on this subject: *"Good health is a process, not an event."*

Once we put our program in motion, moreover, the likelihood of success starts to increase. As new habit patterns begin to develop and become self-reinforcing, and we start to see results, we can move into a *maintenance* phase of change, where the process becomes progressively easier to handle. A conscientious benefits manager in this phase will be constantly monitoring her/his new program, not only for employee compliance but for program effectiveness. S/he will be constantly making adjustments, expanding the scope of whatever program components are most successful, and fine tuning the process so that it is easy and fun for the employees to participate.

Likewise, the individual will quickly be able to identify which elements of her/his change program are working best, and make adjustments in the elements that aren't as effective so that everything they do becomes easier to achieve, mutually reinforcing and progressively more enjoyable. The old adage of *"nothing succeeds like success"* is definitely applicable here; as the person continues to participate, his/her self esteem continues to grow, their state of health improves, and the program becomes an integral part of the employee's lifestyle.

Many of the programs, treatments and therapies that are touted as effectively addressing the various aspects of chronic stress, as described by the Stress Stack, fall under the collective label of CAM. But that begs the question: why should organizations and individuals consider CAM as a primary stress reduction resource?

The Case for CAM – A Powerful Resource to Combat Stress. Were you to do a Web search on the terms "CAM" AND "stress," you would find that there are millions of links that connect those two subjects. A further investigation shows that many aspects of CAM are already widely considered to be major treatment modalities for chronic stress, and in many ways are superior to those made available by conventional medicine. We pay due respect to the scientific advances which have revolutionized conventional medicine over the last several decades, but we know that the recent revelations about their significant limitations, especially in the area of treatment of chronic stress, also deserve our collective close attention.

At the same time, it is apparent that an ever increasing body of holistic health knowledge exists which predates and, in many respects, transcends the framework of conventional medicine. This body of knowledge, combined with those of other peoples around the planet, holds tremendous value in terms of their collective ability to improve the health of America's citizens.

These time-proven therapies and modalities hold the promise of transforming our health care system, its ability to deal with chronic stress, its effect on our economy, and on our society at large. Many leading thinkers in the health care arena, although still in the minority, have begun to recognize this changing dynamic. One of them is Kenneth R. Pelletier, PhD, MD, Clinical Professor of Medicine at the University of the Maryland School of Medicine (UMMC) and the University Of Arizona School Of Medicine. A medical and business consultant to the US Department of Health and Human Services, the World Health Organization (WHO), the Washington Business Group on Health, and numerous major corporations, Dr. Pelletier clearly sees the results of this growth of public awareness of the value of CAM:

"I can't think of any major city where these kinds of services are not offered now. In some states or geographic areas it may be more difficult to find, but it's not absent. There are small and single practices everywhere, as well as major institutions like the Cleveland Clinic or the Mayo Clinic. The demand has been almost entirely consumer driven."

The July 31, 2009 National Health Statistics Reports, *Costs of Complementary and Alternative Medicine (CAM) and Frequency of Visits to CAM Practitioners: United States, 2007*, documented over 83 million Americans spending over $34 billion[i] out of pocket on CAM annually. Additionally, 38.1 million adults made an estimated 354.2 million visits to practitioners of CAM. This rapidly growing embrace of complementary and alternative health care has coincided with a veritable explosion of the population of such practitioners in every state in the nation. The majority of these practitioners are not licensed by the states in which they reside. Despite the apparent lack of supervision, there are almost no reports of practitioner-caused death or injury from these thousands of dedicated professionals. We will discuss the reason why in a later section of this chapter.

Equally important, there is potential for huge systemic health care cost savings by embracing CAM as an integral part of our health care system. For example, the final report of a 2006 Lewin Group study, commissioned by the Dietary Supplement Education Alliance (DSEA), shows that over the period 2008-2012, appropriate use of select dietary supplements would have improved the health of key populations and saved the nation more than $24 billion in healthcare cost avoidance[ii].

To cite just one example from this study, appropriate use of calcium with vitamin D for the Medicare population shows potential avoidance of approximately 776,000 hospitalizations for hip fractures over five years, as well as avoidance of stays in skilled nursing facilities for some proportion of patients. The five-year (2008-2012) estimated net cost associated with avoidable hospitalization for hip fracture is approximately $16.1 billion. This study examined only four nutrients; existing data indicates that much larger savings could potentially accrue by large scale employment of natural products as a complement to conventional medicine.

Additionally, a recent pilot study, conducted by a major state level health care insurance carrier[iii], employed complementary and alternative practitioners (chiropractors) as primary care providers for a large test group. Medical insurance claims from the group dropped by 50 per cent over two years, and in excess of 70 per cent over the remaining five years of the study.

Also:

"Clinical and cost utilization based on 70,274 member-months over a 7-year period demonstrated decreases of 60.2 per cent in-hospital admissions, 59.0 per cent hospital days, 62.0 per cent outpatient surgeries and procedures, and 85 per cent pharmaceutical costs when compared with conventional medicine IPA performance for the same health maintenance organization product in the same geography and time frame[iv]."

Despite evidence like that above, the medical/pharmaceutical/ insurance complex continues to assert that complementary and alternative health care is of limited utility and not cost effective. However, the American consumer maintains that it is a good value for the health care dollars expended.[v]

These are all indications of the growing recognition and acceptance by the American public, and a growing segment of the health care industry, that conventional medical modalities are but one aspect of total health and wellness care. As the cost of conventional medical treatment continues to soar, and its inherent limitations in dealing with issues like chronic stress become clearer, the American public is clamoring for more effective, less costly solutions than those presently offered by conventional medicine.

Given the huge projected cost increases associated with maintenance of the status quo, as outlined in Chapter 2, it is not an understatement to assert that large scale incorporation of complementary and alternative health care at the primary (wellness and prevention) level, as well as in organizational wellness programs, holds the potential of taking full advantage of a vast, untapped resource of wellness expertise that can exert a transformative effect on how health care is delivered in the United States. Effective employment of this same resource can also have a similarly transformative effect on the alleviation of chronic stress for large segments of the American public.

At the same time, such changes offer our government and the citizens it serves an opportunity to directly combat the most direct threat to our future economic well being: unrestrained cost growth in our current health care system due to the increase of diet- and lifestyle-related illnesses caused in large part by chronic stress.

The American people already understand this situation, and its impact on both their health and financial well being. In millions of cases, and with the help of a veritable army of competent, well trained complementary and alternative health care practitioners, they are taking the care of their health, and that of their families, back into their own hands, as they find the solutions offered by the conventional health care system to be ineffective, from both an outcome and cost standpoint.

Institutional and Individual Impediments to Change. However, there are some significant societal, organizational and individual challenges which must be addressed in order for the changes we desire to be successful. There are obstacles within our daily lives which act as sources of counter-conditioning to inhibit change and leave us, individually and collectively, mired in the earlier phases of the change process. Many of these obstacles have become so deeply ingrained in the fabric of our society that they are now considered by many to be 'normal,' and therefore correspond to the precontemplation phase of the change process. On the other hand, I would hope you agree that any behavior or societal norm, no matter how well accepted it may be, needs to be examined and, if necessary, discarded if it contributes to a continuing dysfunction in the society. Otherwise, we collectively would be subscribing to Albert Einstein's definition of insanity, i.e., continually repeating an action or behavior, but expecting a different result each time. The remainder of the chapter will be an examination of those challenges that have acted as impediments to positive change.

Our Technologically Advanced Society: An Institutional Deterrent to Change. As mentioned in the Preface, when I sat in front of my television on July 20, 1969 to watch the first landing on the moon, I did so in an environment which, like many millions of Americans around me, I perceived as offering many advantages and few disadvantages. A very wise man once said that "*change is hard because people overestimate what they have and underestimate* *what they stand to gain*" (Anonymous). There are many reasons why this statement is true but the most fundamental one is that we live in a technologically advanced society. That may sound counterintuitive, but some important, expert research supports this contention. It conclusively shows that the more technologically sophisticated a society becomes, the more averse to risk it also becomes, and therefore the more resistant to change.

This was recently and clearly outlined in an article from the magazine *The Economist*. The author convincingly pointed out that, contrary to conventional wisdom, the major developing countries are now better situated to take full advantage of emerging technological innovations than are the developed Western nations. It cited widespread use of both mobile phones for personal communication in Brazil, and light emitting diodes (LEDs) for residential and business lighting in India as examples of how such countries will be able to both avoid the huge investments in telecommunications and electric power infrastructure that Western nations have made, and position themselves to make even greater, more rapid advances in the future, both technologically and economically.

In contrast, more advanced Western societies, with their huge investment in various forms of centralized infrastructure and bureaucracy, have self-created their own forms of societal and institutional resistance and counter-conditioning to change. These infrastructures and bureaucracies, and the social conditioning they generate, also give rise to large segments of the population who have strong vested interests in the maintenance of the economic and governmental status quo surrounding those segments of our society. We can see this phenomenon at work in many areas of American life, but none more clearly than in our food industry and our health care system.

Our Food Supply: A Change Inhibitor. For example, how may times have we been on a diet of some sort and, when faced with the temptation to eat 'prohibited' food, a friend or family member says something like "*Oh, go ahead. It won't hurt this one time!*" This scenario, and many others like it, is in large part influenced by the nature of our nation's contemporary food supply, and the marketing messages that accompany its choice of products, manufacturing and distribution.

Go into virtually any grocery store and look closely at what's on the shelves and where it's located. A common denominator is that the truly healthy, fresh food (i.e., produce, dairy, meat, poultry and fish) is located around the periphery of the store. Typically, you have to walk through the rest of the store to get to it. In the process, you are intentionally exposed to the location and not-so-subtle associated marketing of the rest of the food in the store, the majority of which is processed food. We've already talked about some of the significant physiological hazards associated with making this type of food the staple of your diet in Chapter 3, so I won't belabor the point here. However, it should be pointed out that another important and detrimental aspect of this food can be the creation of a strong emotional connection (like the one with chocolate!), usually based on the context in which the food is offered. Here's an example from my own family's experience.

When we three siblings were growing up, one of the stores my family frequented was a bakery less than a quarter of a mile from our house. Among other things, this bakery made a cake cookie called "*black and white*," named for its half vanilla, half chocolate frosting. My mother used to buy these cake cookies periodically and bring them home to us as a special treat. To this day, my emotional association with the "*black and white*" is one of love and caring. This connection is not lost on the food industry; turn your television to any station and you'll see commercials which portray similar examples used to market all sorts of processed food products. Obviously, our society's dietary habits are, to a great extent, strongly influenced by emotional factors.

If the food we strongly connect to is a healthy, natural one, the effects can be minimally adverse, or even helpful. Unfortunately, that is not the case with the majority of us. How many people do you know who have strong emotional connections to, say, fruits or vegetables? The influence of processed food, and the emotional association we have with it, can therefore be counted as a strong counter-conditioner to effectively dealing with chronic stress.

Unfortunately, as mentioned earlier, one has only to look at the influence of the funding of the Academy of Nutrition and Dietetics (AND) by food and pharmaceutical companies to see clearly that Big Food and Big Pharma are firmly in the driver's seat when it comes to professional dispensing of nutritional advice. Combine that with a concerted political campaign that has allowed the AND to monopolize 31 states with exclusionary licensing laws, in the process silencing dissenting voices in the area of nutritional counseling, and it is small wonder that the American people are now subject to a new form of 'P.C.' oriented education when it comes to food.

Sadly, this is another example of the 'flat earth' mindset that afflicts much health care-related education in the US today, education that is hugely and inappropriately influenced by Big Food and Big Pharma. If it's not taught in medical school or in dietetics classes, it simply doesn't exist, or is derisively classified as 'quackery.' A prime example of monetary influence within this system was referenced in Chapter 3 with our discussion about caffeinated beverages.

The inevitable and regrettable result for the average American is that, while they're enjoying their fast food meal, they're focusing on the burgers, fries and soda, and certainly not conscious of this pervasive disenfranchisement. That awareness typically surfaces only when they're already firmly ensconced in the disease management system, and by then it's already too late.

Additionally, the combination of strong media marketing messages and the 'advocacy science' used by the processed food and pharmaceutical industries, alluded to earlier and expanded upon later in this chapter, can create confusion in the average American consumer's mind as to what is *truly* healthful. Because food marketing is such a powerful and pervasive force in our society, it acts as an overt deterrent to the search for reliable information about the food products we eat. As a result, we can include this as a counter-conditioning factor to our desire for change, and an impediment to our ability to effectively deal with chronic stress.

Our Health Care System and Chronic Stress: An Overt Impediment to Change. One of the many advantages I grew up with was having a superbly trained family physician, the late Frank Longo MD, who became a treasured family friend. Back in those days, doctors made house calls, and 'Doc' Longo, as we called him, visited us numerous times throughout my childhood in the 1950s and 1960s to assist us with the various ailments I and my siblings dealt with.

Further, I am very proud of the fact that my own stepson is a brilliant young cardio-thoracic surgeon. If I, or any member of my family, were ever involved in a serious accident, I would want them to be taken to the nearest hospital and placed in the care of a surgeon like my stepson. I would *not* want to be taken to a naturopath like me, and be given an herbal remedy for my injuries! We are fortunate to be living in a country where trauma care and acute care is ranked as the best in the world.

However, the huge, Byzantine health care system that supports these capabilities is very much like a dinosaur when it comes to dealing with change. Any small increment of change can ripple through the system and cause tremendous turbulence and controversy. As such, most components of the system, both organizations and individuals, subconsciously resist change; many, out of perceived professional and/or financial self-interest, overtly do so. This includes not only the people who comprise the parts of the system that deliver goods and services, but also those whom the system is supposed to serve. As a result, change is effected very slowly, if at all.

For example, huge portions of the population are still comfortable with the long established health care paradigm of walking into a medical doctor's office, chatting with a cheery receptionist, filling out the newest set of forms, waiting (sometimes for lengthy periods) until their name is called, and then interacting with a comforting authority figure in a white coat, frequently while they themselves are wearing a white hospital gown. This sounds somewhat benign, but look beneath the surface of this process.

Despite the fact that, as demonstrated in Chapter 2, the solutions medical doctors offer are proving to be progressively less effective and more expensive, especially with regard to chronic stress, this care delivery model is clung to almost reflexively, for fear that something will be missed or overlooked, or in the belief that no other options are available. The fundamental reason this system has existed as long as it has is that we, as a society, have collectively chosen to transfer responsibility for the most important aspect of our lives, our state of health, to someone else. We have collectively decided that we are not individually qualified to make important decisions about our own well being, and so we have turned that responsibility over to the medical/pharmaceutical/insurance complex, typically in the person of one of its members, our doctor.

At the same time, many members of the medical community have aided and abetted this collective attitude, both within themselves and within the patients they serve, by both the way they are trained and the way they interact with their patients. From the very beginning of their medical school training, medical doctors are taught to project the aura of both infallibility and power. This is a direct outgrowth of over a century of institutional indoctrination in our nation's medical schools, where the concept of the "*heroic physician*" first arose, was expanded upon, and is now firmly enshrined in the public consciousness. As more and more physicians made their way into their communities, this translated into the societal "*hypnosis of social conditioning*" that, in all matters of health, "*the doctor knows best.*"

As a result, every step of a visit to a doctor's office, as outlined above, subconsciously strips control from the patient and transfers it to the doctor so that, by the time the person in the white coat walks in the door of the examination room, the patient's attitude has typically become one of expectancy, pliability and obedience. This was clearly outlined in a recent *Reader's Digest* article titled *41 Things Doctors Never Tell You*. One doctor was quoted as saying, "*I was told in school to put a patient in a gown when he isn't listening or cooperating. It casts him in a position of subservience.*"

Many doctors also actively discourage their patients from empowering themselves with information outside of the doctor's office. In the same *Reader's Digest* article referenced above, another doctor was quoted as saying, "*Your doctor generally knows more than a web site.*" And when a patient does conduct her/his own research and later has more questions for the doctor, the same doctor's frustrated, internal reaction (but not to the patient) was "*So why don't you get the web site to take over your care?*"

Regardless of how the doctor/patient interaction unfolds, at the end of the visit, when the doctor then pronounces the verdict (i.e., names the disease) and prescribes a remedy (usually a prescription drug, surgical procedure or other medically prescribed modality) to treat the illness, the process theoretically reaches a satisfactory conclusion for all concerned. The patient walks out of the office with the referral or prescription slip in hand, her/his expectations have been fulfilled, the doctor's position of authority has been maintained, and the integrity of the system has been preserved.

Notice I used the word 'theoretically' above. That may be the 'ideal' concept of how the medical/pharmaceutical/insurance complex would like the system to function. Realistically, it doesn't actually work that way. Why not? I mentioned earlier that our nation's health care system is the best in the world with respect to trauma care and acute care. That's directly attributable to the fact that the vast majority of the average medical doctor's education is spent learning pharmaceutical, radiological and surgical medicine.

Unfortunately, however, this information is almost always offered in a context that allegedly demonstrates the asserted clear superiority of pharmaceutical, radiological and surgical medicine over any natural modalities. In contrast to the excellent training offered in the areas of acute care and trauma care, our medical education system is and has long been lacking in the areas of mandatory education of new physicians in CAM and nutrition. That is a likely reason why, in contrast to the widespread American public perception of our health care system as an across-the-board world leader in quality, the World Health Organization has ranked the US #72 on "*Level of Health*" (between Argentina-71 and Bhutan-73) and #37 on "*Overall Health System Performance*" (between Costa Rica-36 and Slovenia-38) [vi].

It is important to note that while virtually every medical school in this country offers *elective* courses in CAM and nutrition, it is a different story when you look at the *mandatory* curricula. A 2007 survey conducted by the Texas Health Freedom Coalition (THFC) of the publicly available (online) information concerning the mandatory curricula of the nation's top 25 medical schools, as rated in 2006 by US News and World Report, disclosed the following:

MANDATORY NUTRITION AND CAM TRAINING AT TOP US MEDICAL SCHOOLS (2006)

MEDICAL SCHOOL	NUTRITION TRAINING*	CAM TRAINING*
1. Harvard University (MA)	2 Semester Hours	None Listed
2. Johns Hopkins University (MD)	None Listed	None Listed
3. University of Pennsylvania	One four week combined course	None Listed
4. University of California–San Francisco	One combined course	
4. Washington University in St. Louis (MO)	One week combined course	None Listed
6. Duke University (NC)	None Listed	None Listed
7. Stanford University (CA)	None Listed	None Listed
7. University of Washington	One two week course	None Listed
9. Yale University (CT)	None Listed	None Listed
10. Baylor College of Medicine (TX)	One six week combined course	None Listed
11. Columbia U. College of Physicians and Surgeons (NY)	Award winning 4 year program	None Listed
11. University of California–Los Angeles (Geffen)	One combined course	None Listed
11. University of Michigan–Ann Arbor	None Listed	None Listed
14. University of California–San Diego	One combined course	None Listed
15. Cornell University (Weill) (NY)	5 clock hours	3 clock hours
16. University of Pittsburgh	8 clock hours	2 clock hours
17. University of Chicago (Pritzker)	20 clock hours	None Listed
17. Vanderbilt University (TN)	None Listed	None Listed
19. U. of Texas Southwestern Medical Center–Dallas	None Listed	None Listed
20. Northwestern University (Feinberg) (IL)	One combined course	8 clock hours (est.)
20. University of North Carolina–Chapel Hill	One combined course	None Listed
22. Case Western Reserve University (OH)	12 week course	None Listed
22. Mayo Medical School (MN)	None Listed	None Listed
22. University of Alabama–Birmingham	50 clock hour course	None Listed
25. University of Virginia	None Listed	None Listed

*The term "combined course" indicates that the nutrition and/or complementary care training was combined with another subject area, e.g., nutrition with gastroenterology. No subject-specific breakout of the course content was offered in the curricula. Sources: online course catalogs for each school listed.

Again, virtually all of these schools offer *elective* training in both complementary and alternative health care and nutrition. However, the data reveal that only 8 per cent of these schools offer any meaningful *mandatory* training in CAM, and less than one third offer meaningful *mandatory* training in nutrition (i.e., information over and above that offered to the general public). In virtually every school, the overwhelming curricular emphasis is on pharmacological, radiological and surgical medicine.

In the preface to this survey, the THFC put the above data into further context:

"... *the overt influence, via substantial funding/endowment, by major pharmaceutical companies on the curricula of these schools virtually assures that mandatory medical education will continue to emphasize pharmaceutical, surgical and radiological medicine at the expense of all else...Further, there are many thousands of dedicated physicians throughout the country who themselves employ nutrition and complementary and alternative modalities in their practices. However, these doctors achieved this largely through extensive self-help and study, in many instances while facing the determined opposition of their own professional organizations and state medical boards.*"

The inescapable conclusion from the above data is that, as a community, the medical establishment does not uniformly possess adequate practical knowledge to pass judgment on the efficacy of, much less effectively employ, CAM and nutrition as a viable alternative or complement to conventional medical care. How could they do so, when they are so minimally educated on the subject? It would be the equivalent of a lay person claiming to be able to perform a complex surgical procedure after having simply read a book on the subject. When compared to the extensive training made available to students in CAM schools, this fraction of medical education is nowhere near enough to equip them to make truly and comprehensively informed judgments about the effectiveness and safety of these remedies/therapies. At the very least, their continual attempts to offer the American public so-called authoritative advice on these subjects call into question their objectivity on this issue.

Moreover, the practical result of this situation is if the patient asks a doctor with a medical education background like those presented above about the effectiveness of any of these therapies, for many of these physicians the default response usually is "*don't use them.*" Part of the motivation for this response may lie in the hesitance of the doctor to admit s/he doesn't really know that much about the subject. But undoubtedly, for many physicians the unspoken but powerful, implied message here is "*I'm the doctor; I know more than you do; don't question my authority and expertise.*" The pharmaceutical industry has recently jumped on this messaging bandwagon in a big way, via a cleverly produced television advertisement; you've probably seen it more than once. In the commercial, the narrator advises "*you don't let your doctor do your job; let him do his!*" In other words, don't question what advice the doctor gives you, s/he knows best.

Think about the above statements for a moment. Those of you who work in an organizational environment know well the value of intelligence, education, clear and innovative thinking, and self-empowerment as ingredients of your company's success. What if your working environment was consistently characterized by thinking like the above, i.e., "*I'm the boss; I know all the answers; don't think for yourself, just do as you're told!*" ? How successful do you think your organization would be if all innovation and self-determination were missing? Might this authoritarian mindset be a major part of why our health care system finds itself in crisis? Unfortunately, that's the underlying philosophy that dominates much of our health care establishment today, a philosophy that, for a variety of reasons, does not serve us well, and is an additional reason why there is resistance to change within our health care system, resistance that significantly impedes the system's ability to deal with the problem of chronic stress.

Paternalism or Self-Empowerment – Which Works Best for You?

Although the concept of the "*heroic physician*" served its purpose in the early 20th century, when the average level of education, and associated knowledge about health, was at a much lower level than it is today, that time is long past. All one has to do is walk into any book store and they will be confronted with shelves full of all manner of books about various health-related subjects. Likewise, go online and do a Google search on any health subject. Depending upon the particular subject matter, there can be literally millions of links associated with the subject. The point is that, today, the availability of information about virtually any health subject is unprecedented in the history of our civilization, and the opportunity for personal empowerment on the subject of health has never been greater.

One would think that our nation's medical schools would have responded to this explosion of information availability by making substantive changes, at both the philosophical and curriculum level, in our medical education system. Some of that has indeed occurred; for example, Columbia University's medical school has incorporated an award winning nutrition program into its curriculum. Regrettably, however, they are the exception rather than the rule. For far too many schools, it is business as usual when it comes to how their new physicians are trained.

As a result, and as demonstrated above, the collective conventional health care professions continue to overly emphasize paternalism in the delivery of health care, depriving our citizens of the empowerment they need to make early, preventive decisions for good health. Over time, a system of gradual disenfranchisement of our citizens has sprung up, creating in the process both a patient population offered poor quality information on preventive health strategies by the medical establishment, and an increasingly disconnected and elitist-minded cadre of care providers. A prominent example of the pervasiveness of that mindset is the use of the term 'peer.'

As I said earlier, I offer all due respect to a person who has undergone the extensive and arduous training of a physician. I definitely want someone with the highest level of training and skills available if I am faced with an urgent, life threatening situation. However, the self-enshrinement of the physician community to a place where the word 'peer' is the sole differentiator that determines whether someone is qualified to even discuss a health related subject is, in my opinion, inappropriate in an environment where so much other, reliable health information is now available. In fact, I consider it downright dangerous to my health if a doctor is even unwilling to discuss information I have, and he may not be aware of, simply because s/he has the initials 'MD' stitched on her/his white lab coat, and I don't.

As a result of this collective mindset, the quality and quantity of information being delivered by those same providers does not begin to match the rapidly changing and growing needs of their patients. Rather than spend their time on devising strategies to match the informational needs of the patient base with its current level of knowledge, large segments of the medical community have apparently elected to write off this crucial component of health care delivery, instead opting for a 'lowest common denominator' approach that serves neither patients nor providers.

This is clearly demonstrated by a recent survey of the practices of family physicians in Ohio. Like most physicians, they spent most of their time treating existing disease, with little or no time spent on patient wellness education. The sicker the patient, the less likely he or she was to receive wellness education. This paradox creates a patient base with growing distrust in the empathy and ability of the providers to deliver them meaningful care, and a provider cadre increasingly isolated from the patients they serve. As long as this attitude persists among these providers, we may count it as an additional major component of the health care system's resistance to change, and a corresponding contributor to its inability to effectively address chronic stress.

"Sicko" Was Right . . . To A Point! As Michael Moore's controversial film demonstrated, a primary factor which contributes to the maintenance of this dysfunctional system is the medical insurance that most patients keep in force. However, Moore's analysis missed some issues which are very important to American society's ability to effectively deal with chronic stress.

The insurance industry has created a dizzying array of codes to describe virtually any medically diagnosed illness. As long as the doctor's diagnosis fits one of these codes, the patient is satisfied (i.e., his/her condition has a label), the insurance company will pay its allotted reimbursement for drugs and services, and the integrity of the system is again preserved. At the same time, for both financial and institutional bias reasons, the industry has collectively decided that most complementary and alternative therapies, which many Americans use as part of their personal stress reduction programs, are of so little use that they do not deserve reimbursement under the system.

Why does this occur? Before a remedy or therapy can be included in an insurance company's repertoire of billable expenses, it must pass the muster of the company's review process. The people involved in this process are primarily medical doctors, financial analysts and attorneys. Their primary motivation is limiting both the legal and financial liability of the company for treatment of a given condition. As such, they rely on the very same type of information that the FDA does when approving a drug.

While this may be a satisfactory system for evaluating drugs and containing costs, an unfortunate byproduct is that virtually no complementary or alternative therapies pass muster, no matter how much empirical evidence there is to prove their effectiveness. If the treatment's 'square peg' of evidence doesn't fit the 'round hole' of the evaluation paradigm mandated by the company, it is not approved for reimbursement.

But there's another, even more compelling reason why most insurance companies don't reimburse for CAM therapies – money. Recall the results of the pilot study, conducted by a major state level health care insurance carrier[vii], and referred to in an earlier section of this chapter. You would think that, confronted with such favorable results, an insurance carrier would immediately take steps to incorporate such treatment into their program on a large scale. But they didn't! The reason given was that, with larger segments of their insured population in demonstrably better health, they would have to lower their insurance premiums. In other words, insurance companies make more money from the treatment of disease, and the resulting sicker insured population, than they do from keeping people well.

The practical result of this is that as long as the health care and insurance communities are dealing with a diagnosable disease, this system can offer at least some help to a patient. However, the effectiveness of the system breaks down when the doctor attempts to treat a patient suffering from chronic stress. There is no insurance code with the text label of stress in the billing system. In a vast number of cases, the doctor can find nothing wrong with the patient. Blood work, EKG, urinalysis all turn up negative. This situation usually ends (frustratingly so for the patient) with physician pronouncements like "*You just need to get more rest,*" or "*When's the last time you took a vacation?*" or "*Maybe it's all in your head.*"

The patient leaves the doctor's office frustrated that no help is available or, worse yet, with a prescription for a sometimes expensive medication, with potentially detrimental side effects, that only offers temporary and symptomatic relief. This leaves open the prospect of that same person returning to the doctor's office, weeks or months later, her/his complaint still unresolved, only to face a reprise of the previous visit, and perhaps the addition or substitution of another expensive, marginally effective prescription. All the while, the employer's health care costs continue to inch ever higher, with no measurable return on the expenditure.

The regrettable conclusions that many people have already reached are that, first, the health care system as currently structured is functionally unable to deliver chronic stress-related care. Second, the ability of the current model of health care delivery to address this issue is medically, sociologically and economically unsustainable over the long term. The combination of rapidly rising costs, systemic inadequacies, and a collective societal mindset of denial of personal responsibility has created a system that does not, and will not, meet the needs of the people it is supposed to serve. Based as it is on the long-ago disproven premise that a person is healthy until s/he demonstrates overt symptoms of ill health, it waits until the damage is done before action is taken.

That is because the indications of chronic stress do not match any current medical diagnosis, and therefore are functionally invisible to the current system until the patient reaches the point where significant damage has already been inflicted. By that time, the need for the patient to access conventional remedies and treatments (e.g., harmful corticosteroid drugs, expensive and invasive diagnostic procedures, or dangerous surgeries) has become a self- fulfilling prophecy.

It is important to note at this point that the answer is definitely *not* to simply declare stress a disease, and then attempt to fit it into the existing care delivery model. It is the model itself that is flawed, probably fatally. And that model can now be counted as one more factor that causes our society to resist change, and diminishes our ability to deal with the problem of chronic stress.

The FDA: Part of the Problem, Not the Solution. The Food and Drug Administration (FDA) is generally perceived by the public as an oversight and regulatory agency. However, it is a little known fact that the FDA is not the impartial arbiter of food and drug safety it portrays itself as, or the public believes it to be. The public perception that has been created over the years of a benevolent Uncle Sam, in the person of the FDA, carefully watching over the health of its citizens, evaporates in the face of the fact that the same food and drug companies who must pass FDA muster also provide funding for the FDA!

This has created many situations where the FDA is actively involved in the promotion of synthetic chemicals, in both the food and drug arenas, over equally safe and effective natural equivalents. For example, the natural sweetener stevia has been marginalized for many years by the FDA in favor of the synthetic substances saccharin, aspartame and (most recently) sucralose. Why? Because synthetic chemicals can be patented, generating years of reliable profits for the 'inventor,' usually a company which the FDA unabashedly calls its 'client.' Only recently has stevia been allowed to make a comeback, but only because a major food company has patented a synthetic equivalent, Truvia. When in doubt, follow the money.

The same logic applies in the drug arena. There are now years of clinical research which demonstrate the pain killing properties of medical marijuana. Yet marijuana continues to be ruthlessly suppressed by federal and state authorities while countless thousands of people annually become dependent, to varying degrees, on powerful, synthetic, expensive painkillers with harmful, potentially fatal, side effects. Once again, follow the money.

As a result, over the years the system of food and drug approval has become rife with potential for corruption. For example, the FDA has on file hundreds of so-called 'conflict of interest waivers,' documents which allow researchers and physicians who have a significant financial stake in the fate of a given drug to actually participate in the approval process. At the same time, FDA employees can move relatively freely among government, industry and academia, creating a truly incestuous relationship among these three groups.

The rationale offered by the FDA and these researchers is twofold: first, the need for a given drug to treat disease is so great that they need to do everything possible to speed the drug to the market. Second, the knowledge of the drug possessed by these researchers is so specialized that only they can adequately determine whether it is safe or not.

Wait just a minute! When you boil this rationale down to its basics, we're allowing people who stand to earn huge amounts of money from the sale of this drug to determine whether it is safe. They're in effect telling us, "*Trust me; I'm a lot smarter than you, so I can tell you whether this is safe. Just ignore the fact that I'll make a lot of money from its approval!*" I remember a very famous 1939 film where a major character was quoted as saying, "*Pay no attention to that man behind the curtain!*"

More to the point, the arrogance of this type of thinking, and the solution to remedy it, has historical precedent in government. In the early 1970s, in the aftermath of the Vietnam War, an eccentric, crusading Wisconsin Senator, William Proxmire, undertook an investigation of the military/industrial complex, specifically the relationship between the Pentagon and the defense/aerospace industry. He coined the phrase *"revolving door"* to describe the phenomenon of a Defense Department official managing the budget of a weapon system one day and, when he retired from government service, going to work for that same defense contractor the next. Proxmire's revelations ultimately resulted in passage of significant legislation reforming the relationship among our government, its employees and the defense/aerospace industry.

Unfortunately, we as a people are currently victimized by the same type of inappropriate relationship between the FDA and the medical/pharmaceutical/insurance complex. To date, no member of the US Congress or the executive branch has stepped forward to remedy this reprehensible situation. A major reason why is that the pharmaceutical industry has the most numerous, highest paid lobby in our nation's capitol. With several lobbyists per Congressman, and millions of dollars of political money at their disposal, is it any wonder why our lawmakers remain silent on this issue?

As a result, no legal firewalls exist between the FDA and the medical/pharmaceutical/insurance complex. The vast majority of FDA decision makers have either worked for food or drug companies in the past or are likely to work for food or drug companies in the future. Many of these decision makers also hold significant financial positions with companies over whose products they exercise approval authority[viii]. As the recent series of spectacular revelations about the adverse side effects of new drugs graphically portrays, it is an obvious and potentially deadly conflict of interest. Although the FDA has recently instituted some reforms, the fact remains that a researcher can still sit on an approval panel for a drug in which he has up to a $50,000 personal financial interest. These restrictions may be waived at the discretion of senior FDA decision makers.

This same problem of split allegiance also affects FDA decision maker attitudes concerning CAM. As a result of their collective background, generated in large part by the medical education system referred to earlier, the institutional bias of FDA decision makers runs very deep. Rather than allow an unbiased, head-to-head comparison of pharmaceutical and complementary medicine, the FDA permits researchers employed by drug companies to publish studies with known design flaws, so long as they are able to either advance the interests of a pharmaceutical company or disparage a competitor in the field of complementary and alternative health care[ix]. A compelling case can be made that this institutional bias within the FDA is intensified due to the additional influence of personal financial interests. This assertion is supported by the conclusions reached by the authors of the JAMA-published study on health care conflicts of interest, referred to in Chapter 1.

As a result, the FDA, with the help of its advocates in the pharmaceutical industry, has been able to use the scientific method to unfairly and inaccurately disparage complementary and alternative health care, to the detriment of both the government and the general public[x]. The revelations of numerous instances of data and study parameter manipulation, and the repeated attempts at FDA rule making to restrict public access to complementary and alternative health care, point to a concerted effort on the part of FDA decision makers to effectively eliminate complementary and alternative health care as a meaningful component of the US health care system.

How does this situation impact the challenge of chronic stress in our society? When our primary government health regulatory agency, the FDA, is dominated by officials who are themselves the product of the "*hypnosis of social conditioning*" that permeates the medical/pharmaceutical/insurance complex, we become saddled with a system that permits only one kind of health care and, more importantly, one kind of thinking with regard to health care. That thinking is the philosophical underpinning of what we know as conventional medicine. Another, less well known name is allopathic medicine. What does the descriptive term "*allopathic*" mean? That depends upon who you ask. The Free Online Dictionary defines "*allopathy*" as "*A method of treating disease with remedies that produce effects different from those caused by the disease itself.*" The Wikipedia definition, which is more expansive, reads in part: "*Allopathic medicine refers to the practice of conventional medicine that uses pharmacologically active agents or physical interventions to treat or suppress symptoms or pathophysiologic processes of diseases or conditions.*"

It is the phrase "*treat or suppress symptoms*" which is, in my estimation, the most important part of the latter definition. It means that, from the outset, the treatment is not designed to address the underlying cause of the condition, but only the manifestations of it. This coincides perfectly with the philosophy conventional medicine has adhered to from its beginnings over a century ago. Don't address the cause of the illness, treat or suppress the symptoms.

The societal ramifications of the persistence of this type of thinking throughout the medical/pharmaceutical/insurance complex, and at the highest levels of government, are staggering. We have been societally conditioned to believe that we don't have to address those underlying conditions at all; we just have to take the right drug or get the right surgery, and we can go back to what we were doing, because conventional medicine has all the right answers. In light of the evidence presented in Chapter 2, I have only one question: how's that working for you?

When you boil this philosophy down to its basics, strip away all the bells and whistles surrounding conventional medicine, i.e., the white lab coats, shiny diagnostic machines, impressive looking medical centers and pharmaceutical manufacturing facilities, the medical establishment is, on a philosophical level, practicing medicine in exactly the same way they did over a century ago! It appears to me that all we have done here is update the trappings and the tools, but we're still delivering a type of care that is for all intents and purposes a century old. More to the point, how effective has this system been in addressing the pandemic of chronic stress in our society? As a matter of fact, it hasn't had any significant effect at all. If it had, we would today not be dealing with the whole host of illnesses whose root cause is stress. Unfortunately, the combination of the financial and bureaucratic interests of the medical/pharmaceutical/insurance complex, and the government officials who support them, creates a huge impediment to change, and therefore to our society's ability to deal effectively with chronic stress.

Scientific Research for Sale.   A primary reason why the above situation exists at the FDA is that it does not possess a large research facility infrastructure of its own. As such, it must rely on the research conducted by other organizations (some government laboratories, but mostly universities, pharmaceutical companies, and food manufacturers) to make decisions on the safety and effectiveness of the products it oversees. In fact, in order to obtain approval from the FDA, a product must undergo expensive research studies that are usually directly or indirectly funded by the parent company that has developed the product. Both the company that is manufacturing and marketing the product to the public, and the research institution for hire, have a huge financial incentive to prove the effectiveness and safety of that product.

Because of the impressive academic credentials these researchers possess, we have been virtually brainwashed to accept without question the accuracy of all these research findings. After all, if Professor So-and-So from the University of Such-and-Such has done a study on this or that subject, well then it must be true because, wow, he has a PhD in that field and I don't! Well, maybe not so much.

At the same time, the overriding business model of our society demands that Big Pharma, like any other corporate entity, manufacture products that earn a substantial rate of investment return for their shareholders. This is not an optional activity; it is a legally enforced fiduciary responsibility. Serious legal penalties accrue to corporations and their officers if this responsibility is not adequately fulfilled. Therefore, they invest huge sums to research, develop, manufacture and market something that is new and patentable so that they can directly profit from their endeavors. They have no choice but to be aggressive about getting FDA approval because of the enormous amounts of money involved.

The irony here is that most natural and healthful products, many of which have been used for thousands of years and sold as supplements, have the FDA standard cautionary warning label implying that it may be unsafe: "*This statement has not been evaluated by the FDA.*" It hasn't been evaluated or approved because there is no financial or political incentive to do so.

Unfortunately, the converse is also true: there is every financial and political incentive to publish studies, no matter how flawed or biased, to portray the asserted superior effectiveness of pharmaceutical medicine over natural therapies. For example, a recent study published in the *Journal of the American Medical Association* attempted to dismiss the effectiveness of vitamin E as a heart-healthy nutrient. What the research report did not tell us was that the researchers used a synthetic fraction of vitamin E, not a more effective and complete natural form, and the study's population was already seriously ill when the nutrient was given to them. How accurate do we think those results were?

Even more recently, a study receiving national media attention allegedly debunked the effectiveness of glucosamine and chondroitin sulfate in alleviating arthritis pain. What the media reports didn't mention was that the study actually only stated that the two nutrients were equal to prescription drugs in relieving pain for people with mild pain, but that they were superior to the drugs for people with moderate to severe pain. How many people with arthritis do you know that have only mild pain? Oh, and by the way, a dozen of the scientists who participated in the study and wrote the press release receive direct compensation from three of the largest pharmaceutical manufacturers who make pain relief drugs!

These are just two examples of many that have occurred over the years. Why does this happen? Once again, follow the money. Government laboratories and university research centers require funding to both operate and justify their existence. If they are not conducting research, and receiving funding for that research, they cease to exist. So if someone from the government or business communities comes to them with a research project proposal, they will rarely think twice about accepting it, especially if the research supports their own organization's point of view.

Interestingly enough, alarm bells are already being sounded about this problem within the health care community. As previously mentioned in Chapter 1, many research scientists are taking steps to distance themselves from corporate sponsors so as to strengthen the credibility of their research as unbiased. No less than the editor of the *Journal of the American Medical Association* has expressed concern about the appearances of impropriety of the relationship between the pharmaceutical and medical communities. A study also published in JAMA by a prestigious panel of authors showed that (no surprise!) medical doctors are just as liable to be influenced by financial and other incentives as the rest of us are.

But perhaps the most damning evidence of the shortcomings of this system were recently revealed in an article released in early 2011 in the *British Medical Journal* (BMJ). The article asserts that "*a large proportion of evidence from human trials is unreported, and much of what is reported is inadequate.*" An accompanying editorial by Dr. Richard Lehman from the University of Oxford and BMJ Clinical Epidemiology Editor, Dr. Elizabeth Loder, characterize the the current state of medical research as a *"culture of haphazard publication and incomplete data disclosure."* This results in much data, which otherwise might negatively affect the outcome of trials of new drugs, being eliminated from reporting. The effect of such practices are all too clear to the authors, who characterize it as *"the evidence we publish shows that the current situation is a disservice to research participants, patients, health systems, and the whole endeavor of clinical medicine."*

Unfortunately, many in the medical/pharmaceutical/insurance complex choose to ignore these warnings, and press ahead with their agenda of continuing to "prove" both the supremacy of pharmaceuticals and the inadequacies of natural therapies. Because they and their corporate sponsors have access to such large amounts of money, they are able to pick and choose what "research" they conduct and, in many instances, what results they achieve.

Unbelievable as it sounds, there are now proven instances of outright research fraud with respect to both sets of research. In the case of pharmaceuticals, research studies cited for a drug's approval were found to be conducted with 'spiked' placebos. In another instance, a major pharmaceutical company was discovered to have actually attempted to entice a health care publishing company to publish several new medical journals, all of whose studies were totally fabricated. In the area of natural health, a 1996 study, widely reported by the media, allegedly 'proved' the ineffectiveness of a popular herb, garcinia cambogia, used in many natural weight management products. What was not reported, either initially or after the fact, was that the study used only half the recommended dosage of the herb, and that it was conducted on behalf of the manufacturer of a major commercial weight loss product.

Additionally, because the medical/pharmaceutical/insurance complex is so wedded to the use of the double blind study for evaluating virtually every health related product, we wind up with studies whose results treat natural products more like drugs. These results completely and repeatedly mischaracterize these nutritional products. For example, studies done on nutritionals such as stevia, Chinese red yeast rice and organic germanium were used by the FDA to either restrict labeling (in the case of stevia), or declare them unsafe (in the cases of Chinese red yeast rice and organic germanium). When examined more closely, the studies have been found to be conducted in such a way as to minimize both the natural products' availability and stated effectiveness with respect to their Big Pharma competition.

This deference to Big Pharma extends into the arena of international trade as well. It is no secret that the international Big Pharma cartel has insinuated its way into the process of 'normalization' sought by the leaders of the Codex Alimentarius Commission, otherwise know as CODEX. If this group of companies has their way, only they and their medical community supporters will be able to manufacture, supply and prescribe natural products above the recommended daily allowance (RDA) in any country, including the US. Following the current model of finding the next big 'blockbuster' drug, these companies will offer only those supplements which guarantee them a steady rate of financial return.

As a result, the small business person who manufactures high quality specialty natural products will be driven out of business. And the consumer will wind up paying many times the current prices for these natural products, if they can buy them at all. Investigative reporter Peter Byrne has written two in depth articles about the inner workings of CODEX Alimentarius that are available on the Smart Publications web site. See the resources section for the links to those articles.

The unfortunate result is that it has become increasingly difficult for the average person to determine whether such research is unbiased, or if it is truly designed to support a predetermined outcome desired by a specific organization, usually with a large financial stake in the results. This type of 'scientific research' is actually a perversion of the original intent of the phrase, i.e., the search for truth. What we witness almost daily with the release of these 'studies' can only be called 'advocacy science.' It is literally a perversion of the scientific method for economic gain. The level of uncertainty about whether any given research study has been conducted free of inappropriate financial influence can thus also be counted as a major impediment to systemic change, and therefore to the ability of the research establishment to effectively address the problem of chronic stress.

The impediment of state level regulation. Since every state has the authority to manage and regulate the actions of its health care practitioners, the focus of attention of many health care professional organizations (e.g., the AMA, the Academy of Dietetics and Nutrition, the American Massage Therapy Association, and their state level affiliates) has increasingly shifted to the state level. Passage of exclusionary licensing laws at the state level has proven to be an effective tool for these organizations to effectively shut out other complementary and alternative health care competition.

Relying on the mantra of 'protect the public,' and preying on the concerns of largely uninformed legislators, they have achieved mixed success. As mentioned earlier, the Academy of Nutrition and Dietetics now has exclusionary licensure over the practice of dietetics and nutrition in 31 states; practicing nutritional counseling without a license in these states is now a crime punishable, in some cases, by arrest, imprisonment and heavy fines.

In contrast, the stated rationale for licensing, 'to protect the public,' has proven to be a chimera. If licensing were an effective tool to promote public safety, we would expect to see significant reductions in injuries and deaths as a result of its implementation. However, the most heavily licensed profession in our health care system, physicians, continues to generate tens of thousands of unintended deaths per year[xi]. The sheer magnitude of these casualties of our health care system was the genesis of the stunning and controversial research paper, "*Death by Medicine*." Authored by Carolyn Dean, MD, ND, and nutritionist Gary Null, PhD, it shows, via over 150 peer reviewed research sources, *that the leading cause of death in America is our own health care system, generating over 780,000 deaths annually.*

In contrast, CAM has been shown worldwide to be among the safest activities known to man. Although the rapidly growing embrace of complementary and alternative health care has caused the conventional health care professions, and some of the organizations above, to sound the alarm, on the basis of safety, as to the lack of professional qualifications of many unlicensed CAM practitioners, their concerns are unfounded, and their motives suspect.

Although the Food and Drug Administration steadfastly refuses to conduct similar studies in this country, risk management assessments in other Western countries have yielded the results in the figures on the next pages. The first, part of a risk assessment study published in Australia, is a logarithmic scale depiction of the risks of various human activities relative to the 1 in a million odds of dying in a crash on a single flight of a Boeing 747 anywhere in the world. The larger the circle depicted, and the closer to the upper right corner of the chart, the greater the risk in relation to the datum event. The second, part of a study published in Canada, depicts the same type of information using the same risk datum point (i.e., a single Boeing 747 flight), only in table form. Both studies were conducted by Ron Law of Juderon Associates in New Zealand.

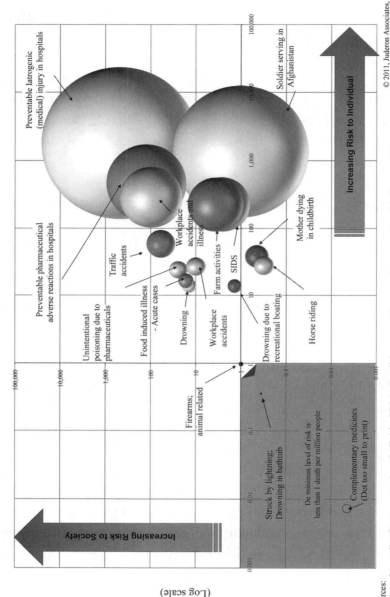

Societal vs Individual Risk of Death in Australia

Bubble size represents individual risk relative to 1 in million (de minimis) approximating the risk of death on a Boeing 747 flight anywhere in the world.

Preventable Iatrogenic (medical) injury in hospitals

Soldier serving in Afghanistan

Increasing Risk to Individual

Preventable pharmaceutical adverse reactions in hospitals

Unintentional poisoning due to pharmaceuticals

Traffic accidents

Workplace accidents and illness

Mother dying in childbirth

Food induced illness - Acute cases

Drowning

Farm activities

SIDS

Workplace accidents

Drowning due to recreational boating

Horse riding

Firearms; animal related

Struck by lightning; Drowning in bathtub

De minimis level of risk is less than 1 death per million people

Complementary medicines (Dot too small to print)

Increasing Risk to Society

Societal Risk: Fatalities per 1 million total population (Log scale)

Individual Risk: Fatalities per million people exposed to risk (Log scale)

© 2011, Juderon Associates, juderon@gmail.com Updated 2011 using latest available data

Sources: Variety of Australian Government and NGO databases and reports.

In other words, a person is significantly less likely to die from administration of complementary and alternative medicines than from a lightning strike.

RISK OF DYING COMPARED TO BEING KILLED ON A BOEING 747 FLIGHT (CANADA)
(DATUM EVENTS ODDS: 1:1,000,000)

UNITS OF RISK PER DEATH	ACTIVITY	RELATIVE RISK
VERY HIGH	ASSOCIATED WITH MEDICAL INJURY IN ACUTE HOSPITALS ONLY	10,348
(<1 PER 1,000)	SMOKING	6,303
"	PREVENTABLE MEDICAL INJURY - (ACUTE HOSPITALS - NZ/ AUS/USA ADJ)	4,085
"	PREVENTABLE MEDICAL INJURY - (ACUTE HOSPITALS ONLY MINISTER'S EST)	3,268
"	PREVENTABLE ADVERSE DRUG REACTION - ACUTE HOSPITALS (NZ ADJ)	1,716
"	CARDIOVASCULAR DISEASE	1,290
HIGH	ADVERSE DRUG REACTION (ALL)	980
(1:1,000 TO	ADVERSE EFFECTS OF PHARMACEUTICAL DRUGS - ALL (USA ADJ)	756
1:10,000)	LUNG CANCER	492
"	CEREBROVASCULAR DISEASE	462
"	BREAST CANCER	311
"	ALCOHOL RELATED (LIVER DISEASE + DIRECT)	277
"	PROSTATE CANCER	233
"	DIABETES	183
MODERATE	ACCIDENTAL POISONING - MEDICINES	46
(1:10,000 TO	INFLUENZA	24
1:100,000)	SUICIDE - PHARMACEUTICAL DRUGS	19
"	FOOD (EST - USA/AUS)	19
LOW	CHOKING ON FOOD/OTHER OBJECTS	8
(1: 100,000	FOOD - HIGHLY PREVENTABLE (EST - USA/AUS)	8
TO 1:1,000,000)	TUBERCULOSIS	3
"	MENINGITIS	1.7
VERY LOW	DATUM EVENT - BOEING 747 (#FLIGHTS- WORLDWIDE)	1.0
(1:1,000,000	ACCEPTABLE RISK FOR CANCER (FOOD ADDITIVES)	1.0
TO 1: 10,000,000)	LIGHTNING	0.25
ULTRA SAFE	BEE/WASP/HORNET STING	0.06
(>1: 10,000,000)	NATURAL HEALTHCARE & THERAPEUTIC PRODUCTS	0.014
"	METEORITE	0.000006

Sources: Extensive search of many Canadian Government, quasi government and NGO websites, documents, databases and research outputs © R Law Juderon Associates 2004. Used by permission. Please see original graph at http://www.smart-publications.com/adrenaline-nation/

In other words, the only thing that is less likely to cause death from natural healthcare and therapeutic products is being struck by a meteorite.

Undeterred by this data, advocates of exclusionary licensing hunt for isolated instances of harm on the part of their complementary and alternative practitioner competitors, and inaccurately portray them as the norm, to attempt to justify their position. Recent information also clearly demonstrates that these efforts at licensing proliferation would result in an increasing burden for cash-strapped state governments[xii].

In reality, the motive for all these efforts is largely financial, i.e., to advance the economic interests of these groups at the expense of their competition. For example, as mentioned earlier, the Academy of Nutrition and Dietetics's web site lists numerous corporate sponsors among the processed food industry as contributing significant financial support to the AND[xiii]. It is not surprising, therefore, that its dietary guideline recommendations substantially reflect the financial interests of its corporate benefactors. The same philosophical bias can be said to exist for the other organizations listed previously.

The practical result of this collective effort is that the American public is denied wider access to competent CAM practitioners, many of whom can offer effective solutions for the problem of chronic stress, all to further the collective interests of a small number of narrowly focused, economically motivated special interest groups, which actively participate in the hindrance of meaningful change.

Mainstream Media: Searching for Truth – Or Profit? Having grown up in a broadcast media family, I have an up-close-and-personal appreciation for its ability to wield influence in shaping public opinion. Properly employed, it can and should be the impartial arbiter of our society, revealing uncomfortable truth when others attempt to conceal it. Thomas Jefferson himself highlighted the crucial role of the press: *"The press is the best instrument for enlightening the mind of man, and improving him as a rational, moral and social being."*

Unfortunately, and in contrast to the role Jefferson envisioned, the modern media over time has also devolved into part of the problem in this arena, with respect to the depth of reporting they do on health issues. Because they hold themselves out to be the communications vehicle of choice for the American people, and because they are relied upon by millions for accurate information, they need to do the best job possible of reporting all aspects of the national health care story. But aren't they already doing so?

In the two examples cited earlier (i.e., the studies about the effectiveness of vitamin E and the supplements glucosamine and chondroitin sulfate), the common element was that, across the board, no major media organ delved any deeper than the repetition of the content of the press releases. Did we see any reporting concerning the apparent conflict of interest with the authors of the latter study? Of course not! Wonder why?

In my opinion, there are several factors at work here. To begin with, many of the people who report health stories are themselves afflicted with the same "*hypnosis of social conditioning*" regarding scientists with advanced degrees that afflicts much of the American public. They are the victims of the 'halo effect,' viewing these people and the expertise their advanced degrees represent as unassailable and, in effect, giving them a free pass on virtually any pronouncements they make.

Additionally, many of these same journalists, by virtue of the circles they move in, come to believe that they are entitled to this level of access to influential people. They view themselves, by virtue of that access and the educational level they themselves have attained, as part of the 'meritocracy' of this country (i.e., the group of people who believe they are entitled to call the shots by virtue of their education and accomplishments). They are not about to jeopardize that position by picking fights with people they view as peers.

Also, many of these same reporters are fearful that if they take too confrontational an attitude toward the stories they report on, they will be denied future access. This is especially true with regard to the investigation of financial connections among researchers, medical organizations and pharmaceutical companies. While media companies such as the NY Times have done some reporting in this area, they have only scratched the surface.

At the same time, many media organs have been complicit in spreading biased and, in some cases, misleading information about natural health therapies. The Life Extension Institute has documented much evidence that major media organs, in conjunction with commercial health interests, have knowingly engaged in a campaign to discredit natural therapies. The previously cited reporting on glucosamine and chondroitin sulfate is but one example of many of this type of biased reporting.

But the final and most important factor is the major reason why such behavior continues. As was recently cited in a major study published in the *Journal of the American Medical Association*, pressure by corporate media interests to keep their sponsors and advertisers happy has the unfortunate effect of suppressing stories that portray a more balanced picture. Why? How often have we seen drug advertising in the middle of TV prime time, or in major magazines or newspapers? The fact is, most of these media organs would now go out of business if they were unable to obtain this source of financial sponsorship. Because much of the media rely so heavily on these advertising dollars from commercial drug and food companies, they are loath to publish or air stories which reflect poorly on their corporate sponsors. As a result, the public is again denied access to balanced, objective information on natural products.

And you don't have to take my word for it, either. One of my friends, an author and health care journalist, characterized the scope of this problem as "... *it's worse than you think.*" He just recently let his membership expire in the Association of Health Care Journalists at his alma mater because of their anti-CAM bias. Apparently, last year they had a CAM authority speak at the annual convention and, as he put it, "*it was like watching a Christian enter the lion's den ... it was ugly.*" On the rare occasions when he himself posted on the forum's board, he was shouted down in vicious terms. As a result, he recently told me, "*you've accurately described their insider mentality.*"

Perhaps the even more convincing information he has provided is the fact that most of the health coverage in the country is now controlled by hospitals and the medical establishment. The media health reporters are being laid off and replaced with spokesmen from the medical community because they're paying for the access and the media needs the money. What was passed off as unbiased reporting before is, according to my friend, "*going the way of the buggy whip,*" and unmistakable information control and censorship is taking its place. Count this as the final impediment to meaningful change, and to our collective ability to effectively address the chronic stress of America today.

As I mentioned at the outset of this chapter, some of these issues are of immense scale. Contemplating them all at once can be a 'gun to mouth' experience for some of us if we let it. But in a participatory democratic republic, the individual citizen is ultimately the most effective agent of change. My goal with this chapter has not been to discourage you, but to empower you with accurate information so you know what the obstacles are, and can avoid having them impede your progress toward constructing an effective stress management program. Speaking of which, to get down to the 'nuts and bolts,' just turn the page.

CHAPTER 8

TEARING DOWN THE STRESS STACK:
ORGANIZATIONAL AND PERSONAL SOLUTIONS

"Natural Forces within us are the true healers of disease"

— Hippocrates

Empowerment: The Key to Tearing Down the Stress Stack. The title of this section may seem a bit counterintuitive, given what we know about health care in this country today. After all, we have been conditioned to believe that when we visit our family physician, we do so with the expectation that s/he will be there whenever we need them, for the rest of our lives, and that they, not we, have all the answers for us with regard to questions about our health. If they don't have those answers, then by definition the answers don't exist. That has been the social conditioning about health care we have received throughout at least the last four generations that have populated this nation. As we have seen thus far, this social conditioning has been shot full of holes by the shortcomings of the very system that created it.

At the same time, if you're an organizational manager or leader, you've also likely figured out that if you or your organization continues to simply shop around the health care insurance market and look for the best existing value, you are doing no more than rearranging the deck chairs on the Titanic when it comes to addressing the problems surrounding chronic stress. No amount of adjusting insurance premiums, increasing copays, or increasing medical savings accounts will address this issue satisfactorily. The old saying of "*if you keep doing what you're doing, you'll keep getting what you're getting*" applies with a vengeance here! What is needed is nothing less than an expansion and redefinition of what is actually covered by company insurance plans in order to reduce corporate health care expenditures over the long term, and allow both organizations and individuals to better address the root cause of most of our country's health problems: chronic stress.

This is not to say that there are no legitimate reasons to continue important parts of the health care system as it exists today. Most of us, our family members, our friends, and our coworkers have had life experiences, such as unforeseen accidents or medical emergencies, which require the very best that the trauma care and acute care segments of our health care system have to offer. When confronted with such a situation, we want, expect and deserve nothing less than the best, most skilled practitioners to care for us. However, when it comes to dealing with chronic and/or degenerative health conditions, including chronic stress, our current health care system falls far short of our expectations, and will continue to do so without meaningful, substantive change at both the organizational and individual levels.

Organizational Empowerment: Successfully Navigating the Process of Change. Whether they realize it or not, corporations and other organizations have a major role to play in this arena. Sadly, most of them have not stepped up to the challenge. Instead, they continue to, in effect, enable the continuation of their own problems. By hewing to a course that, time and again, allows their employees' health to degenerate to the point where much greater expenses are now required, they literally self-inflict their own financial wounds.

Why does this occur? Now that we have drawn back the curtain that has concealed the inner workings of our health care system, as we did in the previous chapter, it becomes patently clear that Big Pharma has a huge investment in people continuing to need drugs, and the processed food companies have a huge investment in people continuing to eat their food. Therefore, these are two institutions which exert a huge drag on altering the status quo. As such, they can be relied on for very little help with changing the situation.

Does that situation need to change? Absolutely! One has only to look at the data I offered in Chapter Two to recognize clearly that we are on an unsustainable course regarding health care in this country. Unfortunately, the proposed solutions emanating out of Washington, from both major political parties, do little more than scratch the surface. They all fail to address the monumental changes that are taking place in the workforce today, and the effect of those changes on the health of our fellow citizens. More to the point of this book, they do not (in any way, shape or form) even begin to address the causative factors that underlay America's pandemic of chronic stress.

As an example, increasing numbers of the Baby Boom generation, financially battered by the succession of crises that has shaken the foundations of Wall Street, are electing to stay in the work force. Since this cohort of the US population remains the largest, it will continue to have the most profound effect on Corporate America's bottom line as it relates to health care for the foreseeable future. Just as the entire US population continues to age, the US workforce will also. Because corporations will have to cover the health care of their employees longer, without profound systemic change, the old paradigm will serve only to continue the vicious cycle of ever rising health care costs, ever increasing stress, and a progressively less healthy, more stressed workforce.

Admittedly, there are some organizations and people who are trying to make changes. Some corporations offer various incentive programs for people to lose weight, stop smoking, or begin an exercise program. For example, the following companies have implemented various wellness-related programs, with measurable success (data provided by the Oregon Department of Health):

- Blue Shield of California saved $8 million in claim costs
- General Electric showed 38 per cent decrease in health care spending
- GE Aircraft reported claims decreased by 27 per cent
- Control Data saved $1.8 million in reduced medical claims and absenteeism costs
- Johnson & Johnson delivered a 30 per cent return on investment
- Tenneco reported 50 per cent lower annual health care claims
- Adolph Coors' estimated health care cost savings of $1.4 million and reported a return on investment from $1.24 to $8.33 for every dollar spent on its wellness program.

Other corporations have taken additional steps toward improving their employees' health. Some offer incentive programs, with rewards like cash and prizes, for losing weight. Still others make fitness facilities available, either on site or via a corporate membership program.

Additionally, there are a handful of companies that even offer very liberal insurance programs which cover a wide variety of health care modalities, including many atypical programs. A prominent example of a company which is a leader in this effort is Whole Foods. You may remember that John Mackey, Whole Foods' CEO, wrote a 2009 *Wall Street Journal* editorial which offered his and his company's perspective on health care reform. In the process he was roundly criticized, I believe unfairly. What he was proposing was a combination of measures, some at the governmental level, some at the corporate/organizational level, to make health care more affordable, effective and empowering. You can read his entire editorial at the link in the resource section. As John Mackey clearly pointed out, it is the concept of empowerment, coupled with that of personal responsibility and management of one's state of health that is the cornerstone of any such successful program.

A big part of the reason companies like Whole Foods remain in the minority is that there are factors which act to hinder change to the status quo. We explored the major ones in the previous chapter. A significant additional factor is how some corporations have historically viewed their health care programs and associated costs. An insightful example of this mindset was shared with me recently by a good friend. One of her acquaintances is a health benefits consultant, whose job is to advise major corporations how to structure their health care plans. In contrast to the logical perception of offering the best health care for the dollar, this consultant admitted that most of his clients ask him to structure their health care plans so they are able to literally push people to the edge of poor health, asking them to maintain an unsustainable lifestyle, with minimal cost to the company.

How shortsighted! While that may work for a little while, in the long run it actually winds up costing a company more, since there are little or no resources devoted to actually preventing poor health. On a larger scale, this mindset boomerangs back onto corporate earnings not only from the costs of the employees themselves, but also from their dependents. The families supported by Corporate America's health care plans are, in aggregate, the next generation of employees. By allowing this shortsighted mindset to dominate corporate decision making with regard to health benefits, these companies are setting themselves up to endlessly repeat this vicious cycle.

Let's take just one example to help prove this case. It's generally accepted that most people develop ingrained food preferences by the age of three. If these food preferences are not healthy ones and continue uncorrected into adulthood, it is very likely that these people will become a cost burden to their employer from their resulting poor health. If the employer devotes no resources to encouraging the employee and his/her family to develop more healthy eating habits, those same family members will likely wind up as part of the next generation of the corporate work force that will become a financial drain on their company's bottom line.

The point of all this is that changing times call for changing measures. When it comes to health care, for its own survival, Corporate America has to begin to take the long view, and not just look at what impacts the next quarterly earnings statement. You're not just impacting the health of your immediate employees, but those in your company's future. We're in a time when all these other factors are in flux. Those companies which choose incorrectly will face a much greater financial burden down the road. Conversely, those which take a genuine interest in their employees' well being will reap dividends far in excess of what the initial investment into preventive care will be.

Individual Empowerment: Living the 'R' Word. The 'R' word in this case is responsibility, as in personal responsibility. As you have seen throughout this book, empowerment, or taking personal charge, is the foundation for an effective stress management program or, for that matter, any effective health care program. Each person must individually negotiate the steps of the change process to ultimately reach the maintenance phase of their personal stress management program. To do so, they must also swim against the tide of the powerful currents of social conditioning that afflict our society when it comes to health care.

The stakes could not be higher. Without sounding too 'preachy,' I also think that we have been both misled and conditioned to believe that the easy way, i.e., taking drugs to mask symptoms rather than addressing the cause of those symptoms, has created the century-long illusion of letting us off the collective hook. It's easier, in a superficial sense, to take a drug than make lifestyle changes like quitting smoking or losing weight. What I'm suggesting here is the expansion of our societal definition of what it means to be responsible for our own health. In order for us to enact meaningful change, at both the individual and societal levels, we must go beyond the current definition of responsibility, which currently includes only finding the right doctor or insurance. We ourselves must start to take a more active role in the management of our own health for meaningful change to take place. But how do we create the foundation for that change in our daily lives? And how do we translate that into a program that effectively addresses chronic stress?

The following is a summary of the philosophical foundation of my professional experience. The information is offered as a set of six principles to use to help guide your personal quest to better manage chronic stress. I will use examples from my practice to demonstrate each principle.

Principle #1: Your selected health care practitioner should walk their talk when it comes to your empowerment. The concept of self-empowerment is the cornerstone of my practice, a concept which I share with each client as we begin to work together to solve their health concerns. The journey we embark upon together with the client can be the most important and exciting adventure of their lives: the journey to improved health. I approach working with them on this journey as teacher, coach, adviser and friend. Unlike medical doctors who have relatively little contact with their patients between visits, I ensure my clients know they can rely on me to personally address their questions and concerns. This is one of several significant differences between the way my practice operates and that of a conventional medical practice. Wherever you are located in this country, I strongly suggest you seek out a health care practitioner who shares this philosophy.

Principle #2: Diet and Lifestyle Are the Primary Determinants of Good Health. As we all well know, a visit to a medical doctor typically involves no more than a few minutes of actual consultation, a review of the symptoms, and the writing of some sort of prescription to alleviate those symptoms. That is NOT what most natural health practitioners are about! As reflected in the information and assessment forms my clients fill out, I am primarily interested in their diet and lifestyle as major determinants of their current and future state of health. If they bring medical test results and diagnoses with them, that's great! I certainly use them as part of my assessment, but blood tests and medical diagnoses are only two of the many pieces of the puzzle that come together to tell the story of a person's state of health. They can anticipate that we will spend a number of hours with them over the next several months putting those pieces of the puzzle together.

An equally important point is that if a client is not willing to implement the diet and lifestyle recommendations I suggest, there really is nothing further I can do for them. As mentioned previously, I believe that "*good health is a process, not an event*," and that includes events like going to the health care practitioner's office. Those events, in and of themselves, will not result in lasting change. If an individual is truly interested in improving their health, the first place they need to look for answers is the mirror. No amount of external help will change a person's state of health if they themselves are not ready and willing to make those changes.

Principle #3 Managing the Stress Stack Requires Change. At the same time, I make it clear that my objective is to help them manage their levels of stress, *not* to construct a strategy which allows them to withstand whatever level of stress they are currently dealing with. Frequently, that stress level is simply unsustainable. Remember that I compared the body's ability to handle stress to a checking account or credit card balance? In many cases, clients come to us with the account overdrawn to the point of bankruptcy, and that situation has existed for many years. They exhibit *all* the manifestations of chronic adrenal exhaustion.

For example, a client in his mid-60s, who was in a very strenuous occupation in the construction industry, came to me for help in dealing with his bone-crushing fatigue. A look at his health history and adrenal salivary tests clearly showed he was chronically overextending himself physically, and was well into the exhaustion phase of the stress response. I constructed an attainable set of diet and lifestyle recommendations and a supplementation protocol, and spent a good deal of time educating him and his wife about the hazards associated with remaining in that situation. Sadly, he chose to ignore that aspect of my advice. Not unexpectedly, he discontinued the protocol shortly thereafter, claiming "*it didn't work for me.*" When last I heard, he was still attempting to overdraw that already empty account.

Principle #4: Change Will Come Gradually. Why do I specify "several months" as the time frame needed to achieve meaningful results? Very simply, because the nature of the changes required for most people dictate that a slow, steady, step-by-step process be followed to return them to good health. When a person shows up at my door, they are usually manifesting stress-related health concerns that have taken, in many cases, decades to develop. It is simply unreasonable to expect that such a set of circumstances will resolve themselves within a matter of a few weeks, or even a couple of months. This is *especially* true when it comes to dealing with chronic stress.

Principle #5: Homework and Self-Study IS Required. Much of what I impart to clients on the initial and subsequent visits is information on how to improve the primary factors involved in effectively managing their Stress Stack. However, as the questions on my forms indicate, I look at a large number of factors before determining how best to help them. I cannot cover all of this information via face-to-face dialogue. Therefore, my practice has generated several important informational flyers that cover some of the most prevalent situations my clients bring to me. They are provided copies of this information, if it is appropriate to their particular health concern, as a part of their consultation. Therefore, it is *their* responsibility to read, digest and (most importantly) *apply* this information while making the necessary changes to their dietary and lifestyle habits. This process reinforces the self-empowerment paradigm.

When applying this principle to your own visit with the health care practitioner of your choice, I suggest you avoid *like the plague* any practitioner, medical or not, who portrays themselves as having all the answers. If they are not willing to discuss information that you bring to your visit, then they have obviously bought into the social conditioning of paternalism. In the long run, that will do your health more harm than good, and certainly provide you with no meaningful resolution of your Stress Stack.

Principle #6: YOU Are Ultimately Responsible for Your Own State of Health. This brings us to the most important distinction between a natural health practice and a medical practice: I *cannot make these changes for the client*. Unlike a medical practice, I do not simply prescribe something for the symptoms so that, when and if they go away, I declare them to be in good health. Pursuing a natural path to good health requires a client to be more than just a passive participant, because the factors that determine a person's state of health are much more than just a set of symptoms.

This journey that client and natural health practitioner embark upon together is a journey of self-empowerment: *their* self-empowerment. The goal is to impart to the client the knowledge, skills and (if necessary) products that they need so that *they* can take charge of their own health and live a healthier, happier, more energetic life. In order for that to happen, the client must participate in this process *actively*. That means taking an active interest in making the recommended changes in their diet and lifestyle, following the recommended supplementation protocols (if any are suggested), and most of all, being *consistent* on a daily basis with those changes. The primary ingredient in their success will be *their* sense of motivation. I have found through experience that the clients who are the most motivated and conscientious are the ones who achieve the best results.

Shifting the Paradigm. What if, based on the principles described above, we could create a ubiquitous shift to a new set of expectations regarding health care in this country? What if we began to create a system where *consumers*, both at the organizational and individual levels, became the primary arbiters of who we saw for health care, what modalities we chose to utilize, and how often we chose to use them? Truly, we would be completely in control of how our bodies were cared for. That is the paradigm that I and many of my fellow CAM practitioners are striving to implement. We believe that *all* health care practitioners need to return to the traditional definition of "doctor as teacher," sharing information with our clients so that they have the tools with which to make their own fully informed choices about their health, and to put in place strategies that allow us to work with them to *prevent* illnesses before they arise.

And make no mistake: we consumers have the ***absolute right*** to demand that from our health care practitioners. When we walk into any health care practitioner's office we are their customers, in effect, *hiring* them. Given the amount of our hard-earned money we spend on health care in this country, almost one dollar out of every five we earn, we have the right to *demand* that they meet our expectations and provide the services *we* want. If they don't, we have the right to seek out *any* type of health care we believe will help us, regardless of the attitude or opinion of the medical/ pharmaceutical/insurance complex or the government.

One of our country's most brilliant inventors, Thomas Edison, presaged this concept long ago with the words "*The doctor of the future will give no medicine, but will interest his patients in the care of the human body, in diet, and in the cause and prevention of disease.*" The future is now.

Education: The Next Step Toward Self-Empowerment. Whether you're an organizational manager or a consumer, let's assume you have moved beyond the contemplation and precontemplation phases of the change process. You've also successfully negotiated the previously discussed "*perfect information*" cognitive hurdle. You're now ready to begin the preparation phase. But perhaps you're a bit overwhelmed at the vast scope of the available information about CAM, and its applicability to your organizational or personal stress management program. Where do you begin?

Fortunately, there are some very credible and easily accessible sources of information that will form the foundation of your knowledge base. To start with, familiarize yourself with the National Center for Complementary and Alternative Medicine (see URL in the resources section). A division of the National Institutes of Health (NIH), the NCCAM site is a valuable compendium of data about all aspects of CAM. It can help you lay the groundwork for what type of stress management CAM resources make the most sense to you and/or your organization.

For those who would like to have a handy printed reference with more detailed information on the various CAM modalities, I highly recommend Alan Smith's *UnBreak Your Health*, now in its second printing. An experienced kinesiologist, print, radio and broadcast journalist, and Amazon-best selling author, Alan has made a career of helping people navigate the forest of modalities that comprise the world of CAM. His book is an easy-to-read guide to the CAM therapies available outside of conventional medicine. Additionally, he has included much of the latest CAM scientific research that validates the safety and effectiveness of the many CAM modalities.

Whether you're an organizational manager or individual consumer, chances are that, once you've delved into the details of the CAM world, you'll want access to resources that allow you to learn more about individual CAM therapies, to share that information with others, and to stay up on the latest breakthroughs. Several health care practitioners and organizations can provide you with top quality information. For example, the *Smart Publications Health and Wellness E-newsletter* can provide you with timely information that can help you stay better informed about the world of CAM. If you're looking for more scientifically oriented information, the professional level newsletter by Smart Publications, *Longevity Medicine Review*, offers online access to the latest in longevity medicine research. See the Resources section for more information about how to access these two informative publications.

Additionally, there are several internationally recognized health care practitioners who offer newsletters on various aspects of the world of CAM. For example, Jonathan V. Wright, MD, who has degrees from both Harvard University (cum laude) and the University of Michigan, has helped advance the science of nutritional biochemistry and nutritional medicine for nearly three decades. Dr. Wright is the author of the best-selling *Book of Nutritional Therapy and Guide to Healing with Nutrition*, as well as other classics in the field. For more than 27 years, he has helped heal over 35,000 patients at his now-famous Tahoma Clinic in Washington State.

Garry F. Gordon, DO, MD(H), is a pioneer in the use of chelation therapy to address a wide range of health concerns including heart disease, neurological complaints and high blood pressure, which may be caused (or worsened) by heavy metal toxicity. Chelation is a medical treatment in which heavy metals are flushed from the bloodstream by means of a chelator that binds to the metal ions. Dr. Gordon received his Doctor of Osteopathy in 1958 from the Chicago College of Osteopathy in Illinois and his honorary MD degree from the University of California Irvine in 1962. Dr. Gordon is Co-Founder of the American College for Advancement in Medicine (ACAM). He is Founder/President of the International College of Advanced Longevity (ICALM) and Board Member of International Oxidative Medicine Association (IOMA). Dr. Gordon has written several books, including *Detox with Oral Chelation*, published by Smart Publications. He is adviser to the American Board of Chelation Therapy and past instructor and examiner for all chelation physicians. As an internationally recognized expert on chelation therapy, Dr. Gordon is now working to establish standards for the proper use of oral and intravenous chelation therapy as an adjunct therapy for all diseases. He lectures extensively on *The End Of Bypass Surgery Is In Sight.*

Marianne Marchese ND, LLC is a clinician, author, and educator. She graduated from Creighton University in 1990 with a B.S. in Occupational Therapy, specializing in neurological and orthopedic conditions, and received her Doctorate of Naturopathic Medicine from the National College of Naturopathic Medicine (NCNM) in Portland, Oregon. Currently, she is professor of Gynecology at the Southwest College of Naturopathic Medicine in Tempe, AZ. Dr. Marchese has had articles and quotes published in numerous national magazines and journals. She is the author of *8 Weeks to Women's Wellness: The Detoxification Plan for Breast Cancer, Endometriosis, Infertility, and other Women's Health Conditions.* Dr. Marchese currently has a bi-monthly column on environmental medicine in *The Townsend Letter.*

Additionally, the *Life Extension Foundation* has a newsletter available that can provide direct access to the latest in CAM news, and the *American Botanical Society* provides internationally recognized research on the properties of herbal remedies. The Resource section has information about how to obtain information from all these health professionals and organizations.

Finally, you can communicate with me directly via links on my Smart Publications page at www.smart-publications.com/books/adrenaline-nation/.

The next step an organizational manager should take is to start researching those insurance carriers available in their state that think 'outside the box' when it comes to coverage of services. There are several carriers that offer a broad range of plans which meaningfully incorporate natural and alternative health care into their menu of covered services. Whole Foods' program, mentioned previously, is but one of many examples. Some offer a combination of a catastrophic care policy and a very liberal medical savings account that allows the insured to reimburse themselves for a wide variety of alternative health services. Still others, like Whole Foods, offer plans where the insured are offered a fixed annual amount which they can spend on virtually any health-related service or product, plus the previously mentioned catastrophic care coverage. Many companies self-fund their insurance programs, in the process offering their employees substantial wellness programs, and incentives for participation. Check with your state's insurance commission for more information about those options available to you.

Complementary and Alternative Health: Expense or Investment?
As mentioned previously, most alternative health care modalities and treatments are not covered by most health insurance plans. The norm for most insurance carriers is that chiropractic, massage, and acupuncture are the only covered CAM expenses, and even those have restrictions with respect to number of treatments and

reimbursable cost. For many people, that means that any alternative health care modalities they choose must be factored into their monthly budget, right along with the rent/mortgage, car insurance, credit card payments, etc. After all, it's just one more in a long list of monthly expenses, right?

Not quite. When we look at the latter categories, in each case there is a payment made for a service rendered, and that is the end of the transaction. Is it the same for complementary and alternative health care? Absolutely *not!* When we follow the guidance offered and implement the dietary and lifestyle changes recommended, the changes in our health are cumulative, progressively longer lasting, and more effective over time. It works in much the same way that a 401(k) or IRA accumulates monetary interest over time. In that respect, natural health care can be considered more of an *investment* than an expense.

Of course, faced with juggling a monthly budget, there is a temptation to classify such an approach to health care as 'too expensive,' especially when compared to the relatively small co-payment made for a routine medical visit. The operative word in the previous sentence is 'routine.' The unfortunate truth is that, if not comprehensively addressed, most health conditions continue to deteriorate and result in *greatly* increased expenses, usually at a time in our lives when we can least afford them. For example, although there are numerous variables that impact the total cost, it is not atypical for the total cost of a heart bypass operation to exceed $100,000. With a typical 20 per cent insurance co-payment, that means that a person recovering from such a procedure, and usually not working, is faced with an unplanned *expense* of over $20,000. In contrast, a one hour consultation with a CAM health professional could typically cost no more than $200, and a monthly cardiovascular-specific diet and lifestyle supplement protocol could cost as little as $75.

Likewise, recall the results of the two studies I referenced in Chapter 7: the Lewin Group study on nutritional supplements and the study that employed chiropractors as primary care providers. Although the cost savings for each study was portrayed in terms of saving money for the health care system itself, these results can also be applied to show how much money individuals can save by living healthier lives.

Do the math yourself. Which is *truly* more expensive, in both monetary and health terms? Obviously, such a decision can only be made on an individual basis. The point we're trying to make is that total good health is truly a case of working on it as we go (a process), not moving from crisis to crisis (an event). An *investment* made now, even if it seems 'too expensive,' can usually help avoid a huge, unplanned *expense* later.

My wife is fond of saying: *"If you can afford to stop at Starbucks® every day on your way to work, you can afford to improve your health now."* The question we all need to answer for ourselves is how important is *now*, and how much do we want to gamble on the outcome of *later*, a gamble which, statistics show, most of us wind up losing. The choice is ours.

Recovering From Chronic Stress: Stepping Back From the Brink. Armed with the tools we have previously created and discovered for ourselves, and the Stress Stack model derived in Chapter 1, let's look at what generally needs to be done to address chronic stress on an individual basis. In the process, we'll also be offering resources that managers can use as the foundation for their organization's stress management program. We'll use the framework created by the "*Day At the Office*" in Chapter 3, insert each stress factor in that workday into the appropriate block of the Stress Stack, and offer potential solutions and/or resources to address each factor. The goal here is to help reduce the magnitude and persistence of each block of the Stress Stack, so that crossing our own catabolic threshold becomes less and less likely.

Please again keep clearly in mind: any effective stress management program needs to address all the factors in order to either prevent chronic stress from reaching a catabolic state, or to recover from a catabolic stress response. While the magnitude and effect of each of these factors will be different for each of us, they will all have an impact on us to some degree; therefore, they must all be addressed in order to achieve the desired results.

In addition, as mentioned in the principles outlined above, we need to exercise both diligence and patience since we are dealing with a hormonally related situation which has, in many cases, taken years to develop. If we're sitting there impatiently tapping our foot as we begin our program, or watching the calendar for the arbitrary date when we can pass judgment on whether it's working, we most likely are not ready to begin. The best way to approach a stress reduction program is with an attitude of watchful optimism: "*I know this is a new program. I accept that I'm still learning about how my body reacts to stress. I'm willing to do what is needed to both increase my knowledge and make meaningful progress. I accept that I may need to make changes in my plan along the way.*"

The wisdom of this approach was graphically demonstrated to me during an airline trip. I was sharing a meal at a layover hotel with a group of my fellow crewmembers, among them a flight attendant from another crew base. When she found out I was a naturopath, she excitedly told me how much the naturopath she had found near her home had helped her with her own health challenges. She also related that, at one point, she had wanted to discontinue the naturopath's program, citing cost considerations. However, the naturopath made a very persuasive case for her to continue. Was she ever glad she did! She freely admitted that completing the program was the best decision she ever made; she felt terrific, and much better than she did at the time that she had wanted to stop.

Unraveling the Stress Stack: Where the Rubber Meets the Road. With the above concepts firmly in mind, let's look at each of the six blocks of the Stress Stack in turn. Because each organization and individual has a different mix of these factors, each will have both predominant and secondary factors to deal with. Some of these will be very challenging for them to overcome, simply because, as we have seen, the society we live in either implicitly or explicitly encourages these same stress causing behaviors. This will ultimately require them to make some very fundamental decisions about who and what they are, what they either expect or need (two very different criteria!) out of their organizational or individual stress management program, and how much effort and resources they are willing to expend to change their situation.

The First Block: Foods and Beverages That Cause Stress. - Moving From S.A.D. to Glad! Recall that I identified several categories of foods and beverages in the first and third chapters which greatly contribute to stress. These were found throughout our "*Day At the Office*," but were most visible in the office break room, during lunch, and when we sat down (or not) for our evening meal.

The first category was caffeinated beverages. I beat up pretty heavily on caffeine in Chapters 1 and 3, and with good reason. It is the most abused substance in our society today; most people are totally unaware of its detrimental effects on the body. You don't have that excuse anymore. All forms of caffeine, including coffee, tea, soda, and chocolate, put our bodies into the fight-or-flight response. They literally drag our bodies back in time, fleeing with A'nath'a down that forest trail to escape the saber tooth. We need to minimize or eliminate all sources of caffeine from our diets; if not, it will inevitably work its wiles on our bodies, with very unfortunate results.

How unfortunate? I briefly worked with a female client and her husband, both in their mid-70s, when we first opened our practice. I was shocked to learn three things about her health history. One, she had undergone a complete removal of her colon (called a "*colostomy*") as a result of the dietary abuse she had inflicted upon her body over the years. Second, despite that rather large wakeup call, she continued to consume at least three pots of coffee per day! She had maintained this habit for over forty years. Third, despite the obviously detrimental effects her habits had on her health, she refused to give up her caffeine use. Needless to say, our professional relationship was rather short!

The second category was artificial sweeteners. Regarding aspartame, or any other artificial sweetener, my advice is simple: *don't use any of them!* While each has its own special way of interacting with the body, they all do harm. This includes Splenda®. As mentioned in the third chapter, although it is marketed as "*made from real sugar*,"the way it is manufactured introduces harmful chemicals (primarily chlorine, which is very antagonistic to the thyroid gland) into the body, much like aspartame does. But what about Truvia®, the newest artificial sweetener, derived from stevia? Manufactured by Cargill®, one of the sponsors of the Academy of Nutrition and Dietetics, it has currently been tested only in Cargill® laboratories. So at this point the jury is still out. However, a conservative approach for now would be to treat it just like the other artificial sweeteners whose history is already apparent. Abstaining from these substances will help to greatly alleviate your body's stress load.

Some people who definitely possess a 'sweet tooth' will, at this point, ask what they can do to satisfy that taste craving. My answer is simple: use natural stevia or xylitol. Despite the FDA, in concert with the big artificial sweetener manufacturers, forcing the relabeling of stevia as a 'nutritional supplement' and not a sweetener, it is a viable and much healthier alternative to these dangerous chemicals. Unless you have a specific allergy or sensitivity to stevia, it will create *none* of the adverse effects that either artificial sweeteners or processed sugars do. Likewise, xylitol can also be used as a sweetener and, when included as an ingredient in chewing gum and toothpaste, has the added benefit of helping to prevent the accumulation of dental plaque.

The third category was processed sugar and white flour. We've talked at length about both the effects of processed sugar and how processed carbs can act as 'rocket fuel for the body,' so I won't bore you with needless repetition. Just know that, to the extent we can cut both of these out of our diets, we are helping our bodies alleviate the load on the adrenals, and therefore our bodies' entire stress response. This includes alcohol, by the way. It is the most highly refined type of sugar we put into our bodies. The more we moderate our alcohol consumption, or eliminate it altogether, the less the stress load on our bodies.

For a different but equally important reason, the same goes for foods containing trans fats. Recall from Chapter 1 that trans fats are attracted to the same cell receptor sites as the 'good' fats like Omega-3 fish oil. Unfortunately, if both are present in the body simultaneously, the trans fats will *always* win the battle to hook up to those cell receptor sites. In effect, trans fats literally starve our bodies of the essential fatty acids they need to support our stress response, accelerating our regression into adrenal exhaustion. So to the extent we can cut these culprits out of our diet, we further decrease the size of this Stress Stack block.

Dealing With 'Allergic' Foods. Speaking of allergies, when I talk about so-called 'allergic' foods, I am actually talking about two different classes of foods. The first are foods which cause either an overt allergic/anaphylactic reaction, such as swelling in the throat, hives, etc. or a reaction due to a genetic inability to assimilate such foods, resulting in major inflammation of and damage to the digestive track. The example of the former that is most familiar to the majority of us is the peanut allergy. Numerous times during my airline career, the crew was required to remove all peanut snacks from the cabin, lest exposure to even the *particles* of peanuts place the passenger in anaphylactic shock.

A dramatic example of the latter is called "*Celiac-Sprue disease*" by the medical community. People afflicted with this genetic abnormality are unable to digest grain foods containing gluten (e.g., wheat, oats, or barley); any attempt to consume these foods results in major intestinal inflammation and discomfort.

However, there is a second, more subtle kind of reaction to foods that are not good for us; some practitioners in the naturopathic community call these 'allergic' foods. I prefer to call the reaction 'food sensitivities.' What do I mean by that? When we consume foods in this category, we are ingesting substances that may not be completely compatible with our bodies. This may be due to the fact that our blood type is incompatible with these foods. Naturopaths Peter D'Adamo Sr. and Jr. have devoted years to the study of the correlation between blood type and diet as a determinant of health. Their best selling book *Eat Right 4 Your Type* contains extensive information on this subject. Please refer to the Resources section for information on their book. Also as a result of our genetic makeup, we may not possess sufficient enzymes to completely digest the foods. I have personal experience with that situation. Despite my love of the taste of fresh cucumbers, I cannot digest them properly. When I order a salad, I always ask that cucumbers be excluded, because "*I like cucumbers, but they don't like me.*" In either case, the result is that our bodies must work harder than normal to break down and absorb these foods.

How can we tell this is happening? Besides our digestive reaction, which can include the obvious manifestations of upset stomach, gas or nausea, our heart is the most reliable indicator. When we are at rest, our heart usually beats at a slower rate than when we are active. This stands to reason; any increase in heart rate is normally precipitated by an increase in the workload of the body. While all foods will create an increase in heart rate simply because the body is expending energy and performing work during digestion, foods to which we are sensitive will result in an even larger increase. So if we ingest food that requires a greater than normal expenditure of energy to break down and absorb, our bodies will signal this by increasing the heart rate. This will also have an impact on the body's stress response, especially if the food is high in glucose. The adrenals will start to secrete increased amounts of cortisol.

The most reliable gage is to first know your own resting heart rate. Then, if eating a given food results in an abnormal increase in heart rate, simply take your pulse. If the heartbeat increases to about 10 per cent or more above your resting rate, that is a good indication that the food is placing stress on your body. While engaged in a program of reducing stress, avoid all foods which create this kind of reaction.

Some people challenge me at this point with variations on the theme of "Aw, you've taken away all the fun stuff. What am I going to eat?" Fortunately, there are some healthful alternatives which, if used conscientiously, can make a huge difference in our energy levels, our sense of well being, and our overall health.

One of the leaders in this arena is a company called Apex Energetics. Based in California, they manufacture and dispense a line of natural products through qualified natural health practitioners. Their continuing education for health professionals is at the top of the

industry.   In conjunction with nationally recognized stress expert
Datis Kharrazian, DC, they have put together a powerfully effective
set of guidelines that I use with all my own clients:

- Do not skip breakfast. Eat a high quality protein based breakfast.
  Each protein portion consumed throughout the day should be
  about the size of the palm of your hand.
- Eat every 2-3 hours. Do not wait until you are hungry.
- Snack with low glycemic index foods such as nuts, seeds, hard
  boiled eggs, etc.
- Avoid all fruit juices and carrot juice.
- Never consume high glycemic fruits or other foods without a
  source of protein.
- Avoid all adrenal stimulants (i.e., the dietary influences I
  mentioned above).
- Eat a well balanced diet consisting mostly of vegetables, quality
  grains and lean meats.

Because of the variability of the availability of foods throughout
the country, I intentionally do not include a so-called diet plan in
this book. However, it is important that I mention one additional
consideration. In the information above, I use the term "*glycemic
index*." What exactly is that? The glycemic index (GI) is a way
of systematically measuring how much the carbohydrates in foods
trigger a rise in circulating blood sugar. The higher the number
(between 0 and 100), the more rapidly your blood sugar will rise
in response to eating that food.

Therefore, as a general rule, choose foods that have lower GI
numbers in preference to foods with higher ones. A good source of
GI information is provided by Thomas Wolever, MD, PhD, Jennie
Brand-Miller, PhD and their co-authors in *The Glucose Revolution:
The Authoritative Guide to the Glycemic Index*. David Mendosa, a
medical research writer and reviewer of *The Glucose Revolution* has
also constructed a website at www.mendosa.com/gi.htm which is

a summary of over 80 studies. The GI data shown there compares each food with eating white bread (a value of 100 on the GI scale). The amount of food consumed is assumed to be about 50 grams (about 2 ounces). These numbers are not absolute numbers, but relative numbers that will allow you to compare foods on the scale with each other.

Don't interpret this as 100 is OK and anything above 100 is high and anything below 100 is not. One hundred (100) is DEFINITELY too high! Try to choose foods in the 70s or lower and go by how your body feels with different foods. This list classifies foods by category (breads, pasta, etc.). Some of these foods you have probably never heard of. Don't worry. This list is a composite of foods tested for their GI value.

If you are relatively sensitive to your body's reactions, you will soon learn which foods give you the right kind of energy, which ones drive you over the limit and which ones drag you down. Use this list as a general guideline. No matter what the GI number, avoid foods to which you are sensitive or allergic.

Applying All This In The Break Room. OK, so how do you, as a manager, apply this in your everyday office environment? First of all, you'll need to start educating your fellow employees about the whys and wherefores of the changes you're suggesting. Given the wide variety of attitudes toward health that people display, and the corresponding place on the spectrum of change they will be, you may expect that you'll get some initial resistance, perhaps quite vocal. However, if you make the information available in this book widely available, and start by offering the healthful alternatives side-by-side with the usual ones, I think you'll be surprised at the response.

Begin by asking your purchasing department to renegotiate your vending machine contracts to include more healthy alternatives in the way of snacks. Most vendors have contracts with several different companies, which each offer healthy alternatives to the standard snacks that currently populate most office vending machines. At the same time, begin gradually decreasing the proportion of sugared and 'diet' sodas in the soda vending machines, substituting instead with bottled water. Yes, I know bottled water has it own set of challenges, but which do you think is better for your employees? An even better alternative is to contract with a commercial drinking water company and start offering water via a cooler. There are several good quality companies out there that offer good quality drinking water.

You can also start to set a good example for your fellow employees, and bring a metal or glass drinking cup or bottle to work with you. Many good choices for these are available at any good health food store. If you purchase a one liter size (equivalent to just over four glasses of water), you'll be able to keep better track of your water consumption throughout the day, and better ensure you're staying hydrated.

If your company contracts with a baked goods company to provide morning break room pastries, ask them to start including more items like bran muffins, and fewer high fat items like doughnuts. Better yet, see if your local organic food vendor can offer a daily delivery of fresh fruit combined with organic baked goods.

The whole point of these collective efforts is to combine your employee educational efforts with gradual behavior modification. As more and more of your fellow employees see others making healthier choices, the effect of social pressure will kick in, and they eventually will climb on the bandwagon themselves and start to modify some of their own behaviors. And if they don't, you will still be better off!

As you continue throughout the day, apply the dietary guidelines offered earlier with each of your meals and snacks. Most likely, the biggest challenge will be at the dinner meal. If you're like most American families, you've become accustomed to the convenience that the availability of fast food offers, to say nothing of the fact that your kids will actually eat it. However, if you want your children to avoid the same health challenges you may face, it's important that you start modifying their behaviors now. Otherwise, you'll be saddling them with some of the same issues you are struggling with. The only difference is now you'll have the additional burden of watching that unfold and knowing you had the means to change it, but didn't. The choice is yours.

The Second Block: Lifestyle Influences - Dialing Back the Stress Meter. Let's take each of the lifestyle issues and factors as they occurred during our day at the office, and discuss some solutions which will help reduce this block of our Stress Stack. As an organizational manager, you can help your fellow employees by incorporating some of these same ideas into your education campaign. As an individual, to the extent you are able to successfully use these tools, not only will you become healthier and more productive, you will also maximize the probability of your future employability.

You'll recall there are a large number of factors. We'll start out by first discussing sleep deprivation. But we'll also include wading through traffic, arriving at the office and sitting down at our work station, and then dealing with our in-basket and associated workload. Then we'll throw in a business trip, and upon returning home, having to deal with household chores, the effect of mass media, and the daily administrative tasks of household management.

Without a doubt, the most important American lifestyle issue is getting adequate rest. I know you've heard it many times before, but the old adage of getting at least seven to eight hours of sleep a night still holds true. The body actually does much of its repair work during the sleep cycle. As mentioned in Chapter 5, the first four hours are spent doing cellular level repair, where the body's resources are used to replenish and repair the damage done during the day. The second four hours are equally important; they allow the mind and spirit to integrate and make sense of the thoughts, events and activities of the previous day. Any shortening of this time leaves you open to a gradual but inevitable deterioration, physically, mentally, emotionally, or all three. Once again, it's those small increments of stress, continually imposed over time, that hold the greatest danger.

At the same time, it's important to be in bed by 10 PM. That may not sit too well with all of you night owls, but there's a very good reason for my saying that. All of us have, at one time or another, experienced what we call our "second wind." We've been awake for an extended period, but for whatever reason we must stay up past our normal bed time. Initially, we may feel tired, but suddenly we get another energy surge, and it seems like we can keep going indefinitely. Ever felt that way? There's a good reason why. As I've said earlier, the human body is a marvelously adaptable mechanism. We all know of situations (e.g., in combat) where people have been able to survive on just a few hours' sleep, night after night. Notice that I said survive. There's a huge difference between surviving and *thriving*. Chronic sleep deprivation places your body in a chronic stress response pattern. Slowly but surely, the effectiveness of your stress response mechanism is eroded. Then one morning, you wake up thinking: "*Why am I so tired?*" By going to bed before 10PM, you will minimize the chances of both getting your second wind, and imprinting a chronic stress pattern on your body.

At the same time, you will be regulating your body's natural Circadian rhythm more closely to what Nature intended, i.e., that you get up and retire with the rising and setting of the sun. As I mentioned in the Chapter 1, the advances of our civilization have made it possible for many of us to literally invert our wake-sleep cycle. The demands of Corporate America dictate that a large proportion of our workforce is assigned to the graveyard shift.

While we usually talk ourselves into believing that we can adapt easily and healthfully to this change, the research says otherwise. Virtually every objective measure demonstrates that this is not a healthy lifestyle. Perhaps the most dramatic example is the cargo plane pilot study on life expectancy that I mentioned in Chapter 3. A five year difference in life expectancy doesn't register powerfully when you're 25 years old. It's quite a different experience when you're 60, up to and including the associated increased health care costs, for both employee and company.

A benefits manager can help with this by acquainting senior management with this important information, and recommending healthful changes to the working environment. For example, setting up alternating shifts can go a long way toward alleviating the effects of this type of work arrangement. This can be especially helpful for parents who already have to split their working hours due to child care issues.

But this discussion leaves out an important factor: what can I use to help me get to sleep and stay asleep, without having to take prescription drugs? There are a number of very well formulated natural sleep aids available on the market today. Any good quality local health food store will be able to offer you an array of products, as well as an explanation of their advantages and limitations. However, a common denominator with all of them is that their effectiveness will be a function of where you are on the scale of stress response. Someone in the alarm phase of the stress response will usually find that any of several sleep aids will be quite effective. As the stress response advances into the resistance and exhaustion phases, though, the effectiveness of a given sleep aid will be determined primarily by an individual's response to it.

You may have to try more than one to find the sleep aid that is right for you. Companies like Health Freedom Nutrition offer several alternatives to address this issue. Refer to the Resources section for their Web URL.

However, let's say you've gotten a good night's sleep, and now you're on the road to work, alertly driving down the highway, and you encounter a traffic jam. What to do about that stressor? This is a prime example of how a shift in attitude can change even the most stressful activities into an enjoyable experience. It's all how you view things; maybe this traffic jam kept you out of a serious accident; tune into relaxing music via CDs or radio. Use your time to listen to audio books on inspirational or educational topics. *Enjoy* your trip.

As a benefits manager, here's another opportunity to help your fellow employees. There are many companies which offer musical or educational products that can assist your employees in better dealing with this type of stress. A call to one of them may help you set up a cross-promotional partnership whereby your employees can enjoy the benefits of musical or educational audio products at a reduced price, and your company can benefit from some positive public exposure by lending its endorsement to those same products.

Likewise, when you're sitting in traffic, you can avail yourself of some healthful stretching exercises. Elaine Masters, a yoga instructor friend of mine, has devised a program called *Drivetime Yoga*, which includes a series of exercises you can do while sitting in traffic in your car. Obviously, these same exercises can also be used in your chair at the office or, for that matter, when traveling on an airplane. See the resources section at the back of the book for Elaine's Web URL.

Once you're in the office setting, what can you do as an employee to minimize the stressors of the office environment? First, it's important that you address your work station environment. For starters, get yourself an ergonomically correct keyboard for your computer. There are many on the market that are available for an affordable price. This will virtually eliminate the risk of repetitive stress injury and the onset of conditions like carpal tunnel syndrome.

Second, check the Yellow Pages for your city and see if there is a furniture store that carries ergonomic office chairs. For example, there's a store called Relax the Back that carries many brands of these kinds of chairs. They may be more expensive than the standard office chairs supplied by your employer, but the investment (there's that word again!) in your musculoskeletal health will pay big dividends in how you feel, your energy level at work, and ultimately how much less you and your employer spend on your health care. This may also present a benefits manager with an opportunity to acquaint senior management with the value of purchasing a suite of such chairs for the workforce as an investment in reducing future health care costs.

Third, take at least a ten minute stretch break out of every hour to give your body a break from immobility. Recall what I said about how the Air Force structured its training. This break from immobility is one of the many benefits. Likewise, you won't be fighting the battle of trying to maintain your attention span while simultaneously struggling against your own body's and brain's reaction to your self-imposed stress. In actuality, taking a ten minute break will help you become a more productive employee!

With respect to de-stressing the work environment, the watchword is mindfulness instead of multitasking. We've already mentioned the value of taking regular breaks, but mindfulness goes far beyond that. There is great value in strategizing the activities of each work day. Try to collect tasks into groups or blocks of the same kinds of activities; do as much of your writing, calling, and meeting together. Cut down on the switching back and forth to the extent practical.

Turning to corporate travel, we've already clearly seen the effect that frequent airline travel can have on our stress levels and, consequently, our health. The most important thing we need to be aware of in this arena is that to the extent we can minimize the impact of the other blocks of the Stress Stack, we can manage the extraordinary demands frequent air travel places on our systems. Beyond that, though, there are several things we can do to better prepare for the rigors of air travel. The first is to get a good night's sleep prior to your flight. Admittedly, that can be a challenge, especially if the preparation activities for your trip occur in addition to your daily workday routine. However, to the extent you can complete those activities without subjecting yourself to a late night prior to the flight, you will be money ahead in terms of your flight being a positive, less stressful experience.

The second thing you can do is abide by the airline's suggested arrival time at the airport so you can negotiate the check-in and security screening processes with as little hassle as possible. Those arrival times are distilled from the collective experience of many travelers before you, so they serve a valuable purpose of not only ensuring you'll be there prior to your scheduled departure, but also of affording you a more stress free experience during this portion of your trip.

If you're traveling internationally or crossing three or more time zones domestically (e.g., on a cross country flight), the challenge of jet lag will be ever present. Fortunately, the world of Chinese medicine offers a very effective technique to overcome this nuisance of long distance travel. Perhaps the best explanation of this technique is offered by Dr. John A. Amaro DC, FIAMA, DiplAc, LAc. A licensed acupuncturist, Dr. Amaro discusses in depth how several simple taps with the blunt end of a ball point pen on the correct acupuncture point can re-synchronize your body with your arrival airport's time zone, allowing you to avoid that "not right" feeling when you step off the airplane. Please keep in mind, however, that this technique will not compensate for the fatigue of a multi-hour international flight. The link to Dr. Amaro's article can be found in the Resources section.

If you're a frequent air traveler, you might take a page from your fellow frequent fliers' and airline pilots' collective experience, and purchase one of the noise reduction headsets that are now available. These have been shown to significantly alleviate the noise-related fatigue of the air travel environment, which is why so many people are now using them. Although the cost per headset averages a few hundred dollars, I think you'll find, as I have, that it's a worthwhile investment in your health, not to mention leaving you much more refreshed at the end of your flight.

While inflight, in light of the very dry air in the cabin, it's extremely important to keep yourself properly hydrated. Try to avoid the temptation to drink caffeinated beverages or alcohol either before or during the flight. The best rule to follow is to emulate the actions of your airline crew. Try to consume at least one 12 oz. serving (can or bottle) of water for every hour of flight. You'll find that you'll arrive at your destination considerably less fatigued, and your body will thank you for the innumerable other benefits you'll enjoy from staying hydrated.

You've now arrived home, and you're dealing with the back side of your day at the office. To overcome the adverse influence of so-called 'labor saving devices' and the culture of immobility they have helped to create, the best solution is to take a lesson from our ancestors. Instead of pushing the buttons on a gadget, push your own button and get moving! You'll recall from an earlier chapter that aerobic exercise is the most effective way to normalize the body's stress response. On a practical level, that means exercising aerobically at least 5 days a week.

Now, by that I don't necessarily mean that you need to go out right away and start jogging, or sweating on a stair climber or exercise bike. In fact, if you're not used to regular exercise that will do you more harm than good. Instead, why not end your evening meal with a pleasant 30 minute walk, preferably with someone whose company you enjoy? A half hour walk at a moderate pace will confer many health benefits, not least of which is the normalization of your body's adrenal hormones. As a result, you'll find that the quality of your sleep will start to improve as well. At the same time, by sharing the experience with someone else, you will begin to create an effective protection against the effect of loneliness on the body's stress load.

We all recognize that the various media devices can sometimes present themselves as an inviting distraction from the rigors of a long workday. As we have already discussed, however, they each present their own source of stress, and thus incrementally add to our Stress Stack. Therefore, it's important to be mindful about our choices of the different media that is easily accessible to us at home.

To avoid increasing our stress load, I recommend we first avoid live news programming, and its attendant emotional content, to the extent practical; if we feel we must 'keep up with the news,' read about it in print or on the Web. It's much easier to avoid upregulation when you read something rather than see it in the format of a live image. Carefully select your TV programs; gravitate toward those that are uplifting or have positive emotional messages. Stay away from violent video games; remember you can literally destroy part of your brain by constantly exposing yourself to this type of stimulus.

And regardless of the amount of take-home work you brought with you from the office, turn off the computer at 9PM, and the TV no later than 10PM. The stimulation of your brain by the energy emitted by the monitors and TV screens can virtually ensure you will not sleep well that night.

Finally, it's important to focus on perhaps the most important of the lifestyle influences, your relationship with yourself and others. Notice that I put *you* before others. You can't expect to have a fulfilling and satisfying relationship with another if you don't enjoy that same thing with yourself. Therefore, it's critically important to take time for yourself in activities that increase your sense of self-esteem and self-worth. Choose a pursuit that nurtures you, like yoga, meditation, art, or writing. It should be one that allows you to healthfully access and express that part of yourself that isn't readily apparent to others. If you are unable to identify such an activity, it's likely time for you to spend some quiet time alone and figure out what *does* affect you in that way. A complementary benefit of this self-examination is frequently a personal reassessment, i.e., answering the question: is what I am doing serving my highest, healthiest purpose?

If you're faced with a long, never-ending string of 'to-dos' at both work and at home, it's time to delegate/prioritize/simplify. What exactly does that mean?

Delegate. Can the task be done by someone else? Don't overlay the decision with emotional content like "*I'm the only one who can do this task this well.*" You've just thrown yourself right back into the same situation you're trying to escape. The watch-phrase needs to be 'don't make perfect the enemy of good.' I hate to clue you in, but *nobody* is perfect, including you! So stop trying to achieve the impossible and relax! If someone else can do the job adequately, let them. You'll likely find that they are able to do a much better

job than you gave them credit for. In the process, with some of
the pressure relieved, *you* will become a more likeable person, to
yourself and others.

Prioritize. Assign a degree of importance, or weight, to *each* task,
without automatically assuming "*it all has to be done right now!*"
Can it be done later, tomorrow, next week, next month? If so, let
it be so. Again, don't pile all that pressure on yourself. Do what
needs to be done now, and don't add additional work, and stress, by
trying to demonstrate you're Superman. You're not; accept it, and
do what you can do and need to do.

Simplify. Treat your work in a different context. How much of
what you do is exclusively geared to keeping the material things
you already have, and how much of it is focused on getting more?
Author T. Harv Ecker, who wrote the New York Times best-seller
Secrets of the Millionaire Mind, offers an innovative idea for dealing
with this trap: want for less. By that he means that if you let go of
the "keep up with the Joneses" mindset, the need for more abates.
Why? Most people tolerate a job to afford a lifestyle. The better
choice is to find a job you enjoy, one that allows you to enjoy the
lifestyle you want, not just in monetary terms, but in terms of
personal freedom and development. Sometimes this means taking
an apparent reduction in the amount of material possessions you
own in favor of a simpler, more enjoyable, less stressful day-to-
day routine. During my airline career, I met several people who
left the corporate world in favor of the less stressful life of a flight
attendant. Some of them had risen to prominence in their respective
career fields. The common denominator, though, was that each felt
that quality of life was more important than quantity of material
possessions. To a person, they each said they were much happier
in their new circumstances. This is true because good health comes
from the interrelationship among the mental, emotional, spiritual
and physical aspects of the universe. Give yourself the freedom
that's more conducive to your lifestyle preference. In the process

of this prioritization, a funny thing frequently occurs. You find out that some of those material things that seemed so important really weren't. So maybe it's time to let them go altogether. The simpler you allow your life to become, the more enjoyable it also becomes.

As you gradually are able to incorporate these ideas into your daily life, you will find that your relationships will become less stressful also. You can help that along by observing a couple of simple principles. First, the old adage of the Golden Rule applies. Treat others the way you'd like to be treated, regardless of how they treat you. Keep in mind that no matter who you're dealing with and when, you're dealing with someone who is the sum of all their experiences up to that very moment. A little compassion, and appreciation for their situation, goes a long way.

Second, take time both during and after work to cultivate meaningful and supportive personal relationships. One of the most meaningful activities that helps build such relationships is eating the evening meal as a family (if you have one), or with friends. Our ancient ancestors clearly recognized that sharing a meal helps build a sense of community. They recognized, as should we, that a strong social network is very important to our overall health and well being.

We should also seek to incorporate these principles into our workplace environment. Of course, we have much less flexibility in being able to do that at the office, so our ability to positively influence others is correspondingly less. This is especially true when dealing with our bosses. If that situation is becoming increasingly unbearable, perhaps that's a signal to you that it's time to start looking for other employment. Nothing is worth sacrificing your health over.

If you are an organizational manager, carefully examine the information offered above. Your ability to apply some or all of it in an employee education program will be a function of your own company's culture and adaptability to change. Simply know that the more material you can impart to your fellow employees, the healthier they will be, and the fewer dollars your company will need to spend on disease management.

The Third Block: Our Own 'Cognitive Filter' - Learning To Think Systemically. As I mentioned earlier, the cognitive filter is perhaps the most influential of all the stressors which impact the human body/mind/spirit matrix. It is the overlay of influences and experiences through which we perceive, interpret and act upon the events which shape our reality. By events, I mean the combination of mental activity, or thoughts, and physical actions which we generate, take or experience throughout our lives. Before, during and after our day at the office, our cognitive filter is constantly at work, so we need to address the context in which it operates. We previously identified both relationships and loneliness in the workplace as prime factors that impact our cognitive filters.

To start with, it's crucial to remember that how we react mentally to stress will determine, in large part, how stress affects the rest of our body. Recall from Chapter 1 that there is some Nobel Prize-winning research conducted by Drs. Guillemin and Schalley which proved that thoughts and mind pictures can be translated into hormone secretions in the body. Since each person's cognitive filter is made up of their unique genetic, biochemical, biomechanical, psychological and spiritual features, the management of their cognitive filter will also be unique. However, there are some common elements that need to be discussed in order to establish a useful framework for everyone.

Perhaps the most important involves a shift in our thought processes from linear to systemic thinking. A friend of mine calls this, quite aptly, 'widening back.' This phrase highlights the necessity of integrating awareness of all the factors that impact one's cognitive filter in order to thrive in a technologically advanced society. So, for example, it's important to be aware that any of the foods we eat, or the lifestyle or toxic influences we expose ourselves to, have a direct effect on how our brains work, how the cognitive filter works, and therefore how we respond to stress. Therefore, to the extent you are able to reduce the impact of those influences, you'll also be able to improve the functioning of your cognitive filter.

Each of the blocks of the Stress Stack will thus have a direct or indirect impact on the cognitive filter. In this section, however, I'll address those proposed solutions that are unique to the cognitive filter and would not be addressed elsewhere.

There are many ways to enhance the ability of your cognitive filter to help you deal with stress. The common denominator with most of them is that they all revolve around having some kind of regular spiritual practice. Now before you react negatively to this statement, please be clear: I'm *not* necessarily talking about religion, or going to church! Having a religious practice is certainly one way of addressing this issue, but it's far from the only one. Whether it's regular church attendance, Scripture study, meditation, using the principles of Abraham or Avatar, being out in nature, whatever it may be, the key is to have a practice that resonates with you, and stick with it. The more that you allow yourself to resonate with the spiritual principles that support you, the more positive your emotional state will be, and the better you will be able to deal with those life issues that can cause stress.

Proven techniques that can help us improve the functioning of our cognitive filter are meditation in its various forms, reframing, and Creative Visualization and Relaxation (CVR). Likewise muscle relaxation/contraction and Bach Flower remedies can be of use. And the NCCAM-recognized systems of Asian medicine and homeopathy can provide meaningful assistance to the operation of one's cognitive filter. Let's look at each of these in turn.

A large and growing body of research has already documented the anti-stress benefits of meditating. Perhaps the best summary of this research is offered by Deepak Chopra, MD, in his 1998 book, *Creating Affluence*:

"There are a number of scientific studies that show the beneficial effects of meditating. Blood pressure comes down. Stress is alleviated. Basal metabolic rate goes down. Insomnia, anxiety, and a number of psychosomatic disorders are relieved and disappear. Moreover, there is increased brain wave coherence, which also improves attention span, creativity, learning ability, and memory retrieval."

Many of these qualities and conditions are not only desirable for the purpose of decreasing stress, but also create the conditions necessary for a person to be more productive. What organization wouldn't want a worker who has the mental qualities listed above!

A common misperception is that meditation is practiced only in the context of a set of religious beliefs. Nothing could be further from the truth. While there are types of meditation that are associated with the practices of Hinduism and Buddhism, as well as other faiths, meditation is truly a non-denominational practice, or can be practiced with no religious belief system at all. The research makes no correlation between the benefits of meditation and a particular religious belief system. So it can be counted as a very effective tool to keep your cognitive filter in shape. See the resources section for more information about meditation.

Reframing is a technique used by both psychotherapists and personal development coaches to help people gain more control over their lives and thus decrease stress. It allows the person to literally see a stressful situation from a different point of view and thus gain a sense of empowerment in that situation. To best learn how to use reframing, one should first either attend a class that teaches reframing, or learn it from a mental health therapist in a clinical setting.

CVR is a new technology that is making great strides in helping people better manage their stress. It combines the best qualities of positive mental imaging and guided relaxation to produce not only clearer mental functioning, but also the following substantial health benefits (information provided by www.newreality.com):

- Increased blood flow to the brain, resulting in clearer thinking, better concentration, improved memory and enhanced creativity.
- A 21 per cent increase in serotonin, which calms the mind and body and creates an overall sense of well being.
- A 25 per cent increase in endorphins, the hormones that flow through your body when you feel happy.
- Better sleep patterns.
- Improved energy levels.

New Reality is a pioneering CVR technology company that has documented the above CVR-generated improvements as part of their product development process. I have personally used the New Reality system and can unhesitatingly say that I have seen improvements in my own health like the ones listed above. CVR is therefore a reliable, effective resource we can count on to help us manage the cognitive filter portion of our Stress Stack.

Muscle relaxation and contraction is also useful in relieving stress, especially the type that arises from repetitive mental or physical work. It consists of sequentially contracting each muscle group (i.e., arm, leg, abdominals, etc.) for several seconds, then relaxing it. I have found this useful when I have been at a task for an extended period, when I have been sitting immobile in an airline seat, or when I haven't been able to exercise and want to give my muscle structure some work.

As mentioned in Chapter 4, a primary influence on one's state of health is the state of the emotions. The stories of Mary and Margie offer stark evidence of the pervasiveness of this influence. But when it comes to actually finding an effective means to positively affect those emotions, conventional medicine offers very limited options. In contrast, the modality of Bach Flower remedies can offer an effective means of addressing virtually any emotional state that contributes to a chronic stress response.

Developed by British researcher Edward Bach in the 1930s, they contain a very small amount of the flower material in a liquid medium. They operate on the principle of conveying the vibration of the plant to help alleviate unhealthful emotional states. Although not recognized by conventional medicine, they have achieved widespread acceptance in the CAM world. As you might expect, these remedies are most effective when they are employed by a trained practitioner. The Bach Centre in the United Kingdom offers a practitioner certification program and maintains a global listing of practitioners who have completed its training program. See the Resources section for a link to the Bach Centre.

The NCCAM recognizes both homeopathy and Asian medicine as discrete systems of medicine. Homeopathy, which originated in Germany in the 1700s, is capable of addressing a wide variety of health challenges. See the Web URL in the Resources section for more information. However, its particular influence on the operation of the cognitive filter is that it can help you alleviate the cognitive component of stress very effectively. Homeopaths use a formulation called "*Rescue Remedy*" as a means of helping a client more effectively deal with the mental and emotional aspects of stress. Rescue Remedy is widely and inexpensively available at most health food stores.

Asian medicine, on the other hand, offers three very effective means of de-stressing one's cognitive filter. The first, Asian herbal medicine, uses a variety of formulations to help the mind and body relax. Some of these are available at health food stores; others must be custom formulated by an Asian medicine practitioner. The second stress alleviator is Asian acupuncture. It is based on the principle that our body conducts energy via discrete bioenergetic pathways, or meridians. The existence of these pathways was proven in 1973 via research conducted in the French hospital system. Use of accurately positioned needles along the appropriate meridians, and on the appropriate points on the meridian, has been shown to be a very effective means of alleviating stress. The third means, Asian body work, encompasses a wide variety of body work techniques that can alleviate mental and emotional stress. It should also be noted that Asian medicine has a very effective nutritional component that can help address the nutritional gap (which will be addressed in detail later in the chapter).

Most states require licensing of Asian medicine practitioners. At present, there is no central information clearing house that offers easy access to a comprehensive list of these practitioners. An intelligently structured Google search will help you find an Asian medicine practitioner in your area.

Since everyone's cognitive filter is unique, it's important that each individual find one, or a set, of these solutions that works for them. To the extent we can accept and embrace the natural, learning from experiences in the process, we can alleviate, if not eliminate, the cognitive filter as a source of stress. Conversely, to the extent we allow frustration or other negative emotion to eat away at the body, we enhance the impact of the eventual emotional component of stress and, eventually, illness.

The other aspect of caring for our cognitive filters is to care for the vessel that contains it, our own bodies. Each of the other blocks of the Stress Stack impacts our bodies directly, but one element that is usually left out is the biomechanical component. It is very important to take proper care of ourselves in this respect also, because all of the solutions for the other blocks of the Stress Stack will affect our biomechanical system to some degree. Therefore, keeping it healthy with good biomechanical preventative maintenance like chiropractic, Rolfing, massage, or other quality body work can go a long way toward minimizing, if not eliminating, the effect of this factor on our cognitive filter. I have included web URLs for each of the three modalities listed above in the Resource section, with links to how you can find a reputable practitioner.

If you're an organizational manager, you're likely scratching your head right now and wondering how these resources can help your bottom line. I invite you to 'widen back' and think about it for a minute. To the extent that your employees' cognitive filters are de-stressed, they will be able to more easily access the portions of their brains that handle judgment, creativity and decision making. And to the extent those functions are optimized, each employee, from a customer service rep to a corporate executive, will be able to contribute more meaningfully to the success of the company. I recognize that this benefit does not lend itself to quantification, but the principles that support it are contained in countless well researched books about good management, so I would hope that any forward thinking manager would recognize that correlation.

The Fourth Block: The Nutritional Gap - Closing the Gap with Nutrition and Hormone Balancing. The most critical idea that must be understood in addressing the nutritional gap is that your dietary intake has a direct and predominant impact on the functioning of your endocrine/hormonal system. This, in turn, has a direct impact on your body's stress response. In other words, the old adage of *"you are what you eat"* is 100 per cent accurate. So how do we address this important block of the Stress Stack?

The first step is to avoid all those foods that actually cause stress. I know we discussed this important factor earlier; the reason I'm repeating it is that each of those foods also increase the nutritional gap by depleting some of the very nutrients we most need for dealing with stress.

For example, caffeine will greatly deplete vitamins B and C, which we'll talk about more in a moment, as well as key trace minerals. It also exhausts the adrenal glands. Artificial sweeteners deplete key brain chemicals that help the brain better deal with stress. Processed sugar and white flour products cause exhaustion of both the adrenals and the pancreas, diminishing the body's ability to respond to stress and hastening the onset of adult diabetes.

On the positive side, I can't emphasize enough the value of eating a plant based, whole food diet for starters. Fruits and vegetables just offer so much value in terms of the wide variety of nutrients they contain. Also, as mentioned earlier, we need to have a regular source of good, high quality protein in almost every meal. The reasons are two fold: first, protein offers the building blocks of the amino acids we need for many of the body's energy producing and rebuilding processes. But there is a little known but equally important second reason: protein helps our bodies to better control and use the glucose that is in our bloodstream from other foods, allowing us to maintain a more even energy level throughout the day.

Additionally, we all need to be taking a comprehensive suite of nutritional supplements that contains all the key vitamins and minerals we need for stress response support and health maintenance. There are many good products on the market today, and make no mistake; quality matters. I discovered probably the best, most descriptive motto pertaining to this issue in a health magazine in Tampa, FL while I was still an airline captain. It said, very simply, "*Your body is the vehicle you drive through life. Why not drive a Cadillac?*" So it stands to reason that the fuel you put in your 'Cadillac' should be of the highest quality.

But how do you determine that quality? Perhaps the most important way is to ensure that as many as possible of the vitamins and minerals that you ingest come from *natural* sources. The way you can tell that is very simple. On the back of each supplement bottle, many vitamins are listed as the d, the dl or the l forms. The d for is the natural form, whereas the dl form has a combination of natural and synthetic forms, and the l form is 100 per cent synthetic. For reasons discussed earlier in this book, I strongly advise you to buy supplements which have as many of the d forms of vitamins in them as possible! Keep in mind that there are cases, especially with respect to trace minerals, where the only form available is either the dl or l form. As long as the majority of the ingredients are natural, you should be OK.

It's also very important to ensure that those key nutrients which support a healthful stress response in our bodies are available in adequate quantities. Ideally, we should be getting these from the foods we eat, but for a variety of reasons I've discussed earlier, most of us do not. If you were to do a chemical analysis of the adrenal glands as compared to other tissues, you'd find that they contain 25 times the vitamin C concentration of the next highest tissue. So it's critical that adrenals which have been under chronic stress get adequate vitamin C, much more than the daily minimum. Obviously, the ideal would be to obtain those from natural sources, such as fruits, green vegetables, or herbs. But because of the factors we talked about earlier, most of us don't get enough from our diets. So I recommend supplementation with at least 3,000 milligrams (three grams, or to bowel tolerance, whichever is less) of vitamin C every day. Ideally, you should take C in small doses throughout the day, but if you can't, get it into your body anyway you can.

Second, the adrenal hormones cortisol, DHEA and aldosterone are derived from the cholesterol that the liver manufactures, so it makes sense to provide the liver with the best raw material possible. That raw material is Omega-3 fish oil. Again, I recommend getting that from eating cold water fish, such as salmon and tuna, several times a week. But if you're concerned about the media stories about mercury contamination of fish, fish in your area is too expensive at the market, or you just don't like the taste of fish, then I suggest you supplement with pharmaceutical grade fish oil, taking at least 1,500 mg a day. You'll also get the additional benefits of better heart and brain health in the bargain.

Third, the effectiveness of the central nervous system portion of the stress response depends greatly on the availability of adequate amounts of all the B vitamins. Once again, ideally I would recommend a healthy diet as the primary source of the B vitamins, especially since each of the vitamins in the B complex is spread out among so many foods. However, the limitations of our society's food supply again make it important that we supplement with a good quality vitamin B complex to address this portion of the issue.

Finally, the portion of the stress response that manages the body's mineral balance needs sustenance as well. So I recommend taking a good suite of quality trace minerals to support that portion of our stress response mechanism.

Contrary to popular perception, this is where an organizational manager may be able to exert their most positive leverage in helping their fellow employees, at little or no cost to their company. Here's an innovative way they could do this. An organizational manager could enter into a cross-promotional partnership with a natural products company, whereby the natural products company could offer preferential pricing and ordering terms to the organization and its employees in return for some favorable advertising exposure. This would allow the organization's employees to obtain quality natural products of their choice at below market prices, in return for the corporation's endorsement of those products.

As part of my own desire to serve my clients, in conjunction with Health Freedom Nutrition, I have developed three nutritional supplements that address all of the above stress support factors. Called *National Defense*, these products contain natural, herbal relaxants that can help the body better deal with the mental and emotional components of the stress response. Please see www. hfn-usa.com for more information.

I mentioned earlier that there is a direct correlation between nutrition and hormone balance. There are many such interrelationships that apply to the hormonal system. In my opinion, the most important involves helping the adrenal glands recover from chronic, protracted stress. This is true because, as I mentioned in Chapter 4, the functioning of the adrenals impact the operation of virtually all the other endocrine glands. Once the adrenals have been balanced, it is much easier to address issues with the other parts of the endocrine system. As such, we should generally start with the adrenals when we are rebalancing this important bodily system.

At this point, please be very clear that there is only so much you can do for yourself to accomplish this important task. While we all can definitely incorporate the advice for self-help that has been offered thus far, this particular piece of the stress management puzzle is *not* a DIY project! You therefore have to locate and procure the services of a qualified holistic or integrative medical practitioner with training and experience in dealing with adrenal hormone balancing. If you are an organizational manager, this may be the most important health care service you can make available to your company's employees.

Since most of these practitioners' services in this arena are typically not covered by conventional health insurance, you can help in four ways. First, you can locate such a practitioner near you or your workplace. There are several resources to help you do this. If you're looking for an integrative medical doctor, the American Holistic Medical Association maintains a listing of its members who have expertise in the area of stress management. If you're looking for a naturopath, two organizations, the American Association of Naturopathic Physicians, and the American Naturopathic Medical Association, both have resources that will allow you to locate such practitioners. Another highly trained resource, the clinical nutritionist, can be located via the International and American Association of Clinical Nutritionists. The previously mentioned chiropractors and Asian medicine practitioners, as well as Ayurvedic (i.e., East Indian) medicine practitioners can also help close this nutritional gap. Individual companies, such as the previously mentioned Apex Energetics, also maintain lists of trained practitioners in your area with stress management skills. I have included a list of organizations which maintain a practitioner data base, along with contact information, in the Resource section. Keep in mind, however, that some very reputable practitioners do not belong to these organizations, so I recommend that you check locally as well.

Second, you may ask your insurance carrier to expand/incorporate alternative/integrative medical services into the reimbursement criteria of the health care savings account. Third, if that is not possible (and that may frequently be the case!), you may arrange for a favorable, discounted fee directly from the practitioner you choose for all employees using the practitioner's services. Fourth, you can arrange to have the practitioner offer their initial assessment services at the corporate offices. This will have the dual positive impact of making the services easier to access, and empowering your fellow employees with more information to make smarter health decisions.

Why is this assessment so important? In extreme cases, the body almost completely loses the ability to control the stress response, so it needs help in regaining control. The first step in accomplishing this is to ascertain exactly in what stage (i.e., alarm, resistance, or exhaustion) the stress response mechanism is operating. In turn, this gives the practitioner a direct reading of the health of the adrenal glands and provides the foundation for recovery. Once again, don't try to do all of this by yourself! Accurate assessment requires the help of a trained professional.

There are several reliable assessment techniques available to natural health and integrative medical practitioners to assess the health of the adrenals. Two of the most common and effective are salivary hormone and computerized bioenergetic assessments. Each of these has distinct, associated advantages and disadvantages.

Salivary testing is useful for adrenal and reproductive hormone evaluations because the information gathered is real time, as opposed to blood testing, which reports what has already happened. Also, salivary testing can be time phased, throughout a day, week or month, which is especially valuable for hormone evaluation. On the other hand, the accuracy of salivary testing can be easily compromised if the test samples are not properly handled and shipped in a timely manner.

Bioenergetic assessment has the advantage of not requiring the delivery of any bodily fluids. Its mechanism of evaluation is to measure the body's, and associated organ systems', energy field at discrete points associated with the acupuncture meridian system. This allows a measure of not only the individual energy states, but the discernment of patterns of energy misdistribution, hyperactivity and weakness. However, bioenergetic assessment is only as accurate as the combination of the information programmed into the device, and the skill of the practitioner in using the device and interpreting the results. Additionally, it's important to note that bioenergetic assessment devices should *never* be used as a tool to diagnose disease! If you are evaluating a practitioner for your own use or that of your company (and I always recommend you do so!), always ask that question as a part of your process. If a practitioner claims to be able to use their device for diagnosing disease, run the other way! They are using their device in an illegal manner, and could subject you and/or your company to legal jeopardy from the FDA.

Regardless of what type of assessment tool is used, a competent practitioner can construct an accurate picture of what is going on hormonally in a client's body, and help the client build a workable plan to better deal with, and eventually recover from, the effects of chronic, protracted stress. Since there are thousands of possible and potentially complex scenarios that could occur, based on each individual's personal Stress Stack, I won't try to offer general advice about this phase of stress management here. Rather, I would encourage you, whether as an individual or a manager, to actively search for well qualified natural health or integrative medical practitioners who can address the assessment piece of the stress management puzzle in a professional manner.

The Fifth Block: Toxic Exposure - Cleansing Is Easier Than You Think. Continuing to refer to our day at the office, we encountered several toxic influences. Factors as diverse as personal grooming products, our office building, the electromagnetic environment inside it, and the packaging of food products can exert unhealthy influences. Likewise, food fertilizers, the air travel environment, and smoking also add to our personal Stress Stack.

All of us want to look our best each day, especially when we are interacting with others in a professional environment. So not using personal grooming products is generally not an option. However, you'll recall from Chapter 3 that as little as a trillionth of a gram of any substance is enough to start a low level hormonal reaction in the body. Is it any surprise, therefore, that chemical exposure, regardless of the individual dose, is a major stressor in our society? When we take into account the cumulative nature of this exposure from examples like the ones we discussed earlier, the ever growing toxic stress load we are imposing on ourselves becomes increasingly apparent.

To address this part of our Stress Stack effectively there are a couple of important things that we need to do. First, be more aware that these influences exist, and do your best to avoid them. So, for example, I now make it a practice of not spending any more time refueling my car than necessary. Also, to avoid the effects of accumulating aluminum chlorhydrate in my body, I've stopped using antiperspirants and instead use plain deodorant. To the extent practical, I also use all natural skin care products. There are many good product lines available; the important thing is to avoid products whose ingredients are synthetic chemicals.

Since we spend about one third of our lives at work, we can't do much directly about the construction of our office building, or the environment inside it, but we can do something about how long we stay in it and how we interact with that environment. For starters, get out of the office during lunch, preferably to get some exercise. Stay in the office only as long as you absolutely need to be there. This gives us all a new perspective on the true value of "*face time,*" doesn't it?

Additionally, when the weather outside is comfortable, try using a new discovery called "Earthing" to help your body's own electromagnetic field re-harmonize itself with that of the Earth. It involves nothing more than taking your shoes off and sitting for 30 minutes with your feet in contact with the ground. It doesn't matter whether it's the bare earth, grass, or even concrete. The important thing is that your body is in direct contact with a conducting surface that will allow your own electromagnetic field and the Earth's to interact. Research conducted by holistic cardiologist Stephen Sinatra, MD, co-author of the book *Earthing*, has shown that daily "Earthing" will help the body rid itself of both stress and various ailments. The resource section has information about how to procure Dr. Sinatra's book.

To protect against those airborne "critters" that wander around office air conditioning systems, several things can be done. First, get a personal air ionizer that can sit on your desk, and use it every day. It can filter out germs and bacteria from your immediate environment. There are several effective models, some of which can be purchased on Amazon for less than $10. Once again, this offers a manager an opportunity to help their fellow employees. Contact the manufacturer and ask them if they can offer a corporate discount for their ionizers. You can use the same kind of cross-promotional partnership arrangement you used for the audio products company. You may also be able to do that with some of the other products I suggest. Contact the company in question for details.

Next, you can further defend yourself against infection by washing your hands frequently, especially if you have just eaten, gone to the restroom, or have sneezed into them. Third, avoid contact with people who are known to be ill. Fourth, give your body an additional layer of protection by using Health Freedom Nutrition's *National Defense* daily to provide the best possible nutritional support to combat illness.

In Chapter 3, we saw how the electromagnetic environment of our corporate workplace can invisibly but significantly impact our health via long-term exposure to various sources of electromagnetic radiation. But that merely begs the question: how do you combat these stressors? First, it's important to know that those sources which are both discrete and in our immediate work area can be effectively neutralized. There is some cutting edge technology available that can minimize your exposure to radiation from desktop and laptop computers, cell phones, PDAs and the like.

A visionary company called GIA makes a passive electronic chip which adheres to most any electronic device. It's been proven to neutralize the vast majority of this type of radiation. As I'm writing right now, in front of my computer, I have GIA chips stuck on my monitor and computer tower. I also use them on my laptop and, of course, my cell phone. See the Resource section for information on how to obtain the GIA products.

Please note, however, that I just said these chips neutralize the *majority* of cell phone radiation, not all of it. So it's important that you, as a manager, ensure that the information on cell phone radiation presented in Chapter 3 is effectively disseminated to all your employees, along with an admonition to use a wired headset (not wireless) along with the phone as a means of further minimizing exposure. To shield yourself from Wi-Fi related radiation, the folks at GIA have come up with an additional device that can help. It's a pendant called the GIA Life Pendant, and can help shield you from the effects of environments like Wi-Fi networks.

When we look across the huge spectrum of products which have been created over the last century to help make our lives easier, there is a common denominator for many of them: they are made of synthetic chemicals derived from petroleum. While these plastics, cleaners, machine parts, etc. all serve productive functions, many of them also have an unintended side effect: when introduced into the body, even in small doses, they mimic the effects of certain hormones, especially estrogen.

As such, as we discussed at length in Chapter 6, they have been collectively assigned the name *xenoestrogens* ("xeno" being a prefix meaning "from a foreign source"). The impact of these substances is that, once they are introduced into the body, they migrate to the same receptor sites on our cells as do the real estrogens produced by our own hormonal systems. Once there, they act as a multiplier of the effects of real estrogen, including the tissue proliferation associated with uterine, breast, and other forms of cancer.

Again, the question remains: how do we avoid or combat the effects of these harmful substances? For starters, I recommend that you only consume water from glass or metal bottles. While it has been recognized for a while that soft plastic bottles and other such containers slough off molecules into water and food, at one time it was thought that polycarbonate containers did not pose that risk. However, additional research has uncovered the fact that anything other than glass or metal containers pose this risk of incremental chemical contamination. Second, completely stop heating foods in containers made from those same materials. The processed food companies still insist in packaging their products in these containers, so you'll have to remove the food from the containers before heating.

Speaking of which, I highly recommend that you *not* use a microwave oven to heat your food, period. Microwave radiation is extremely destructive to the nutritive properties of food, and should be avoided whenever possible. In an employment context, that may mean that you not bring foods to work that require heating in the company microwave. Better yet, ask your benefits manager to see about purchasing a small convective or toaster oven instead.

Additionally, as we have discussed earlier, the chemicals we have used on our fruits and vegetables did not increase the nutritional value of the food, but were used to grow bigger, better looking crops that sell well at the market. In the process, we have progressively grown less and less nutritious food, and paid the additional price of chronically exposing ourselves to continuing doses of these same chemicals. The answer? Eat organic.

While I recognize that organically grown produce is more expensive, when you weigh out the pluses and minuses, in the long term it is actually *less* expensive. By that I mean that by consuming organic foods now, to the extent your personal budget allows, you will delay or avoid the effects of this type of toxic chemical exposure later, and thus lessen the likelihood that your body will tip over into the disease state.

We all know that, at some time or another in our lives, many of us *do* have to interact with the conventional medical community and thus take some sort of prescription drug. However, as we discussed in an earlier chapter, another category of toxic exposure is *definitely* prescription drugs. It's important that we emphasize here that we're not advocating ignoring a medical doctor's advice. We're barred by law from doing that. However, what we *can* say is that to the extent we can keep ourselves healthy, by following the other advice we offered earlier, we can avoid putting ourselves in that situation in the first place.

I spent a great deal of time in Chapter 3 describing the toxic exposure to which frequent travelers and airline crewmembers are exposed. Here's how to combat that set of stressors. To shield yourself from the various types of radiation, use the GIA Life Pendant discussed earlier, or something similar. It can help shield you from both the effects of high altitude radiation and those of earthbound devices like Wi-Fi networks.

Regarding exposure to biological toxins carried by other passengers, to the extent you have a nutritional gap, you will be less able to fend off the immune system challenges that being around everyone else's illnesses will generate. So it's important for you to both eat healthfully and take therapeutic doses of the vitamins and nutrients that we mentioned in the previous section as being the best for helping to fend off the effects of chronic stress.

Finally, while on the ground, do your best to avoid situations where the aircraft is being cleaned with chemical cleaning solutions, and with the doors open, exposure to the fumes from the jet fuel-powered auxiliary power unit. A single exposure to this environment would not normally be harmful. Again, it is the *cumulative* load of each individual exposure, multiplied by hundreds of times every year that subjects people to significant, comprehensive toxic stress.

Please understand clearly that I'm not advocating that you avoid air travel altogether. Remember, I earned my living in that industry for over 16 years, and the air travel industry performs a valuable service for billions of people around the globe. But be aware that airline travel can create health challenges, and that you do have the power to alleviate their effects with proper planning and intelligent use of the available tools.

We've already run through all the reasons why we should avoid nicotine. Just like the foods listed in Chapter 1 under Dietary Influences, nicotine results in the activation of part or all of the body's stress response. Bottom line: nicotine should be completely avoided as a part of a stress recovery program.

Toxic Influence Removal: Some New Solutions. One of the most important services any natural and alternative health practitioner can offer her/his clients is the effective removal of toxic substances from the body, otherwise known as detoxification. This is usually one of the most critical steps in the process of helping a client back to good health. In particular, the removal of toxic heavy metals such as mercury or cadmium can greatly contribute to the restoration of health, in some cases very rapidly.

There are many different ways of detoxifying the body either externally (e.g., colon hydrotherapy, electrolytic foot bath, far infrared sauna) or internally (e.g., nutritionals, cleanses, or herbal/ homeopathic therapies). While offering a client the convenience of completing the therapy at home, many of these internal therapies had the disadvantage of generating varying degrees of uncomfortable side effects. That is, until now.

Recently, Waiora, a forward looking, cutting edge nutritionals company partnered with a brilliant young biochemist to offer what is proving to be the most effective and easy-to-use detoxification product ever discovered. It is called, quite simply, *Natural Cellular Defense*. This innovative product, available in the form of easy-to-use liquid drops, employs a special form of zeolite, one of about a hundred naturally occurring combinations of volcanic ash residue and sea water that possess an extremely strong negative charge. Via a patented process, this zeolite is cleaned of all naturally occurring toxins so that its detoxification properties can be safely employed in the body.

Once inside the body, this particular zeolite's cage-like structure latches onto and 'imprisons' the strongest positively charged particles it can find. These also happen to be the very same toxic heavy metals mentioned earlier. Acting via a process called "*chemical affinity*," the zeolite will remove the strongest positively charged toxins, then the next strongest, etc. until the heavy metals are eliminated. The elimination process occurs very simply, through normal urination. Obviously, it is critical that a client drinks plenty of water during this time. Once the heavy metals are removed, it goes after the chemical toxins, working in the same manner. An additional significant benefit is that *Natural Cellular Defense* can also help to rebalance the pH of the body, moving it from an unhealthy acid to a healthful alkaline pH.

What is the evidence supporting its effectiveness? Clinical trials at a major medical teaching center showed conclusively that significant increases in heavy metal urinary excretion occurred while using *Natural Cellular Defense.* This increase was observed between 4 and 15 days after starting to use the product, depending upon the degree and length of heavy metal exposure. Equally exciting, and unlike other internal detoxification therapies, *Natural Cellular Defense* creates virtually NO side effects! The worst observed has been a mild 'energy slump' lasting no more than a few days. As you might expect, this new detoxification technology has taken the health care world by storm. Check the Resources section to find out more about *Natural Cellular Defense.*

The Sixth Block: The Trigger Factor - Stepping Back From the Brink. You'll recall from Chapter 1 that the trigger factor is one of the least acknowledged factors that impact our health. That's because most people think linearly about their health. They assume that a single incident is responsible for their descent into ill health. In most cases, however, their bodies have literally been teetering on the brink of ill health for an extended period of time. The event I call the Trigger Factor simply pushes their bodies over the edge, as opposed to being the proximate cause of their illness. This situation is usually created by continual indulgence in stress-causing behaviors, creating a set of conditions which set them up for triggers such as accidents to exert their powerful influence.

The primary means of avoiding the emergence of the Trigger Factor in your life is to minimize the influences of the other five blocks of the Stress Stack. If we embark on a strategy to decrease the magnitude of each of the other five factors, we make it much less likely that the trigger factor will ever intrude into our lives. Simply, if we are able to decrease the influence of all the other factors, the likelihood that any or all of them will actually trigger a catabolic stress response is *greatly* decreased. Actions taken to decrease the effectiveness of each of the other factors therefore have a synergistic effect on the effectiveness and sensitivity (or lack thereof) of the Trigger Factor.

What Exactly Did We Accomplish? If an organizational manager, or an individual, employs the knowledge and tools I have imparted to you throughout this book, you will inevitably see the magnitude of each of the factors which contribute to chronic stress *decreasing*. We have addressed each of the factors contributing to a catabolic stress response with effective, countervailing behaviors and strategies. This is indicative of the desire and need to address all the factors we can in order to either *prevent* chronic stress from reaching a catabolic state, or to recover from a catabolic stress response.

While the magnitude and effect of each of these factors will be different for each of us, they will all have an impact on us to some degree; therefore, they must all be addressed in order to achieve the desired results. By embracing this comprehensive strategy, we are afforded nothing less than the opportunity to *finally* take the future of our health into our own hands and start to make constructive, meaningful and long lasting changes. That, in turn, will have measurable, long lasting impacts upon both our workforce's productivity and cost.

Connecting the Dots: An Integrated Strategy. Of all the insights I have shared with you, perhaps most important is your understanding that chronic stress is a holistic phenomenon. In this 'fast food'-oriented society with its emphasis on easy, quick fixes, we tend to gravitate to anything that seems rapid and simple. However, recovering from the effects of chronic stress is neither. The conditions that have created your Stress Stack have, in most cases, taken years to develop to their current state. In order for you to recover from them, they *all* need to be addressed. This may, in some cases, take a period of several months to accomplish.

We've all seen the ads and promotions that tout this or that product or piece of equipment that claims to be able to reduce your stress within 30 days or so. Beware of these 'quick fix' solutions, claiming to quickly relieve your stress in a matter of days or weeks. They may be able to stave off the symptoms you are experiencing, but the underlying processes will still be busily at work and, in time, will inevitably overwhelm those quick, easy fixes. Only when you embark upon a plan, like the one above, to comprehensively address all of the factors in your Stress Stack will you begin to effectively and permanently solve the problem.

The required solutions don't stop here, however. There are some pressing state and national level issues that must be addressed if the challenge of chronic stress in the workplace is to be overcome. Turn the page to find out how you can help to overcome them.

CHAPTER 9

AVOIDING THE COLLISION

*". . . I see in the near future a crisis approaching that unnerves
me and causes me to tremble for the safety of my country. . .
Corporations have been enthroned, and an era of corruption
in high places will follow, and the money of the country will
endeavor to prolong its reign by working upon the prejudices of
the people until all wealth is aggregated in a few hands and the
Republic is destroyed. I feel at this moment more anxiety for the
safety of my country than ever before, even in the midst of war."*

— Abraham Lincoln

*"We have merely scratched the surface of the store of knowledge
which will come to us. I believe that we are now, a-tremble
on the verge of vast discoveries - discoveries so wondrously
important they will upset the present trend of human thought and
start it along completely new lines."*

— Thomas Edison

At the Crossroads. In Chapter 7, I identified the impediments to
change at all levels that must be overcome to effectively address
our nationwide pandemic of chronic stress. Chapter 8 offered
extensive resources and solutions for you to address chronic stress
at the individual and organizational levels. But as I pointed out in

Chapter 2, there are larger societal issues that must also be addressed if we are to facilitate and implement meaningful change. In order to do that, we must tie together the societal factors we first identified in Chapter 2, and correlate them with the impediments to change we identified in Chapter 7. Only then can that meaningful change be implemented.

Never before in our history have we simultaneously experienced the convergence of the quotes above from Lincoln and Edison. We are indeed enjoying breathtaking advances in virtually every field of science and technology, advances that hold the promise of fulfilling Edison's vision. However, as Lincoln feared, we are also now burdened with a governmental, business and societal structure that, for primarily parochial and financial reasons, is fiercely resistant to any change of the status quo.

As a result, we are at a crossroads in our society with respect to its ability to further withstand the detrimental effects of chronic stress. The choices we make in the coming few years will literally determine the future course and sustainability of American society. The sad fact is we are literally burning ourselves out, both as a society and as individuals. At the same time, our society is undergoing extraordinarily rapid change to the point where, according to recent estimates, the body of knowledge in the area of health is doubling every five years. So it's only fair to ask the question: is our society truly keeping up with and adapting to this explosion of knowledge, or is that new knowledge serving only to tighten the grip of those who wish to stubbornly maintain the status quo?

Although the definition of a good job in the United States has almost always included health care benefits, the manner in which that health care is administered, delivered and paid for over time has, quite literally, priced our workforce out of the global labor market. We can carp all we want about the inadequacy of Third

World working conditions and health care systems, but when the cost of a car is increased by $1500 at GM due to health care costs alone, as has occurred in the recent past, we've got a big problem.

A major part of that problem is that our nation at present offers our citizens little in the way of stress management/reduction resources. The stakes for not addressing that shortfall could not be higher. The demonstrated correlation between productivity increases and health care costs, absent a preventive component, has an otherwise prosperous society teetering on the edge of bankruptcy. If the effects of chronic stress are not addressed soon, they will continue to detrimentally ripple throughout our society, ultimately causing significant, perhaps irreparable, physical, mental, emotional and economic damage to increasing numbers of our citizens. At the same time, via the continued and pervasive paternalism that permeates virtually every aspect of our health care system, we are gradually eroding the most effective means of addressing this crisis: the individual empowerment of our citizenry to have unfettered access to an objective body of information that will help them improve and sustain their health.

While it can not be quantified by any financial statement, I believe that every American citizen's single most important asset is their health. This concept of the invaluable nature of health has been a constant throughout the ages. The Roman poet Virgil, author of the epic tale *The Aeneid*, said "*The greatest wealth is health.*" Revered social activist Mohandas Ghandi believed "*It is health that is real wealth and not pieces of gold and silver.*" And the American poet Ralph Waldo Emerson stated, very simply, "*The first wealth is health.*" And while it is also not codified in the Declaration of Independence or the Constitution of the United States, I believe that every American's single most important right is the right to bodily integrity, which includes the right to decide for themselves how their bodies are cared for and what they will put into their bodies. One of the signers of the Declaration, Benjamin Rush, who was also George

Washington's personal physician, presaged our current dilemma over two centuries ago. He bemoaned the lack of a constitutional provision protecting the American citizen's freedom of choice with regard to health decisions as follows:

"Unless we put medical freedom into the Constitution, the time will come when medicine will organize into an undercover dictatorship to restrict the art of healing to one class of Men and deny equal privileges to others; the Constitution of the Republic should make a Special privilege for medical freedoms as well as religious freedom."

As the direct result of not implementing Dr. Rush's advice, our society has been literally hypnotized into believing that only one system of health care is effective, safe and even legal. Truly, conventional medicine has organized itself into an undercover dictatorship that has usurped the right of the American citizen to obtain health care assistance free of parochial influence. Although we have not followed Dr. Rush's advice, I still fervently believe that health freedom of choice is an inalienable right in our country. It is a cornerstone of the foundation of our free society. Ultimately, whoever controls your health care controls you. So the most important question that any American citizen must ask themselves is: who do you want controlling your health care? I have often wondered how that question might actually be answered in the society at large. If a national polling organization were to ask just one question, *"who is responsible for your health care,"* how many do you think would answer *"me?"*

As mentioned earlier, I also think that we have been both misled and conditioned to believe that the easy way, i.e., taking drugs to mask symptoms rather than addressing the cause of those symptoms, has created the century-long illusion of letting us off the collective hook. It's easier, in a superficial sense, to take a drug than make lifestyle changes like quitting smoking or losing weight. Sir Ken

Robinson, PhD, author of the best selling book *The Element*, has some insight as to why this attitude has become enshrined in our collective consciousness:

"Much of Western thought assumes that the mind is separate from the body and that human beings are somehow separate from the rest of nature. This may be why so many people don't seem to understand that what they put into their bodies affects how it works and how they think and feel. . . The rate of self-inflicted illness from bad nutrition and eating disorders is one example of the crisis in human resources."

As a result of this collective mindset, we are now face to face with the enormous costs that we and our children will have to bear if meaningful change of that mindset is not implemented. But how do we create the foundation for that change in our daily lives? And how do we translate that into a program that effectively addresses chronic stress?

The Ripple Effect: Socioeconomic and Sociological Consequences.
This regrettable situation has arisen due to a number of influences that have acted on our health care system for the better part of a century. As outlined in Chapters 2 and 7, the combination of the infrastructure and bureaucracy of our technologically advanced society, an embedded, paternalistic health care bureaucracy, a medical/pharmaceutical/insurance complex desirous of continual expansion of its power and influence, regardless of the societal and economic costs, and a food production industry that emphasizes profit over true health, has distorted the ability of the system to deliver meaningful health care solutions to our citizens. This especially applies to the challenge of delivering meaningful stress-related care.

A Strategy for Success: How to Alleviate Chronic Stress in the US.
As outlined in Chapter 8, a central part of the solution is, indeed, the
individual empowerment of both our citizens and the organizations
of which they are a part through access to reliable information about
both the causes of chronic stress and the means to alleviate it. But
in order for this to be accomplished, a coordinated effort on the part
of both government and business, devoid as much as possible of
parochial economic influences, must also be successfully mounted
and prosecuted.

One of the pleasures and privileges I have enjoyed in my capacity
as chair of the Texas Health Freedom Coalition has been the ability
to work with a group of extremely talented, dedicated and well
educated professionals in the natural health arena. While there are
many on the THFC executive committee who fit this category, my
business partner, colleague and friend, clinical nutritionist Radhia
Gleis, CCN, MEd, PhD is among the top of this group. She has
collaborated with me on many projects, one of the most meaningful
of which has been the writing and publishing of a policy paper titled
The Cure to 'The Sorry State of American Health'. This policy paper,
which I referred to in Chapter 2, was titled to play off the cover
story of a late 2008 issue of *Time*. It was submitted to the Obama
administration's health care task force, as well as to the lieutenant
governor of the state of Texas, and the health committees of both
houses of the Texas legislature. Unfortunately, the undue political
influence of the medical/pharmaceutical/insurance complex on both
the federal and state governments ensured that virtually none of its
recommendations were accepted. *The Cure* addressed many of the
issues we have discussed throughout this book, as well as others
which also directly impact the collective set of actions which must
be implemented to address the problem of chronic stress. I want
to acknowledge Radhia for her contribution, via *The Cure*, to this
portion of the book.

It is apparent that, for an integrated stress management strategy to be successful, these recommendations must be implemented at every level of society, starting with our schools. But none of them will be successful unless significant numbers of our fellow citizens take action and become involved in the process. I will discuss the ways you can help at the end of this chapter.

Recommendation #1: Enact federal legislation to require much more in depth health and wellness education at every level of our educational system. The curricula for this education must be as devoid of commercial interests as possible. Virtually every major processed food manufacturer can trot out so-called scientific evidence to show that their foods are healthy. As we have seen, however, thanks to the unforeseen side effects of the Bayh-Dole legislation, science is now for sale in this country, making virtually every scientific study suspect in that regard.

Accordingly, at the direction of the President, the US Department of Education and Health and Human Services, in conjunction with the US Surgeon General's office, needs to convene a blue ribbon panel of independent health experts who can address the data objectively. Every member of this panel must be thoroughly evaluated for potential conflicts of interest. Any expert who has ties to either Big Pharma or Big Food should be excluded.

This panel should also be empowered to construct new dietary guidelines for the American people, based on both the objective nutritional needs of our population and the actual state of our food supply, as opposed to the current guidelines, which are skewed in favor of both Big Food and Big Agriculture. The *Food Pyramid* (and now, the *Food Plate*) has been used without success since 1979 to offer nutritional advice to our citizens. The results have been an epidemic of obesity, diabetes and chronic and degenerative illness in this country. It's time to throw it all out and start with a clean sheet of paper. Achieving this goal would help clearly define for the public the correlation between consumption of certain foods, and the relation of lifestyle factors, to the incidence of the leading causes of death in this country and, in turn, the correlation of those causes to the incidence of chronic stress.

Additionally, the panel should be charged with identifying measures that will help better educate families on self-help measures they can take to improve the health of all family members. This can include creating new incentives for states to develop health care education programs which more heavily emphasize the value of complementary and alternative health care in this context. It should also include a strategy for prosecuting a campaign to educate and empower the public with useful and effective information on complementary and alternative health care, with emphasis on self-care and childhood education as an additional means of preventing the ten leading causes of death. The panel's recommendations and results should be reported to the Secretaries of Health and Human Services and Agriculture for action and implementation.

Recommendation #2: As a condition of certification and/or receipt of any form of federal assistance or grant, the US Department of Health and Human Services must require mandatory, objective education on diet, nutrition, intelligent use of natural products, and complementary medicine in all US medical and osteopathic medical schools. It is time to end the 'flat earth' mentality in academic medicine. The mindset that if it isn't taught in medical school, it isn't worth knowing is a complete fallacy. It is a well known fact that the curricula in medical schools are dominated, if not completely controlled, by the advocates of pharmaceutical medicine and their silent benefactors, the major pharmaceutical companies. In their ground breaking new movie, *Thrive*, co-executive producers Foster Gamble and Kimberly Carter Gamble reveal that many medical schools offer only 2 ½ hours of nutritional training in their entire four year curriculum. This tracks closely with the survey data presented in Chapter 7. Small wonder, then, that new physicians receive little reliable information about natural and alternative therapies. It's just not taught or, more likely, intentionally suppressed at the behest of Big Pharma and Big Food.

Again, the results speak for themselves. If our medical education system is so superior, then why are eight of the top ten leading causes of death in this country still diet and lifestyle related? Where is the education and training that would allow physicians to address these pressing health issues? Unfortunately, the medical education system is still structured to chase the health care horse after it has left the barn, not to construct a sturdy pen to keep it from escaping in the first place. As a result, we truly do not have a health care system in this country; we have a disease management system, one that at a philosophical level has remained unchanged for over a century.

At the same time, the entire field of nutritional science has galloped ahead over the last several decades, with hundreds of new and effective products available to help people substantially improve their health. There are numerous well-educated individuals in the nutritional sciences field who can provide new physicians with well researched, useful information to allow them to offer their patients viable natural alternatives for dealing with their health challenges. Our medical schools should be seeking these professionals out, instead of locking them out.

Recommendation #3: Reform the Food and Drug Administration.
As mentioned earlier, in the early 1970s, Senator William Proxmire publicly decried and exposed the 'revolving door' that then existed between the Pentagon and the defense/aerospace industry. His efforts spurred Congress to enact tough new legislation that erected legal firewalls between government Defense employees and the industry they oversaw.

No such firewalls exist today to protect the public from the effects of conflict of interest regarding FDA employees and the companies whose activities they oversee. Advocates of the status quo defend the current system by pointing out that, in many cases, only a few people possess the knowledge to make informed judgments on the safety and effectiveness of a particular food product or drug.

If that is true, then we as the public should be asking why that food or drug is being approved in the first place. In an ostensibly democratic society, do we truly want to turn control of our most precious asset, our health, over to any group that is so insulated from public influence? Given their track record to date, do we really have enough confidence in them that they should be able to dictate to us, as opposed to the other way around? I think not.

As such, just as in the Defense Department, legislation should prohibit former FDA employees from employment by a pharmaceutical company or any of its non-profit affiliates, with whom they have had official government dealings, for a period of one to five years after leaving government service. The law should specify strict new limits, over and above what is already being observed, on:

- The ability of FDA employees to exercise regulatory authority over pharmaceutical or food companies, for whom they have worked or will work, immediately before or after government service.
- The ability of government-paid researchers or consultants to participate in the approval process of drugs or food products in which they have any direct financial interest.
- The ability of FDA decision makers to determine the validity of health claims for drugs, foods or natural products without taking into account the financial interests of the researchers in the outcome of the research being used to make the decision.

The length of the prohibition would depend on what degree of oversight the federal employee has exercised, and where s/he worked while employed by the government, or acted in a consulting role for the government. That time interval has worked well since the 1970s in the defense/aerospace industry; the health care industry should be treated no differently.

Further, an FDA Reform Act needs to mandate that the FDA fairly and uniformly enforce the existing definitional provisions of the Food, Drug and Cosmetics Act as they pertain to drugs, foods and dietary supplements. Currently, that section of the act reads as follows:

The term "drug" means (A) articles recognized in the official United States Pharmacopoeia, official Homoeopathic Pharmacopoeia of the United States, or official National Formulary, or any supplement to any of them; and (B) articles intended for use in the diagnosis, cure, mitigation, treatment, or prevention of disease in man or other animals; and (C) articles (other than food) intended to affect the structure or any function of the body of man or other animals; and (D) articles intended for use as a component of any article specified in clause (A), (B), or (C). A food or dietary supplement for which a claim, subject to sections 403(r)(1)(B) and 403(r)(3) or sections 403(r)(1)(B) and 403(r)(5)(D), is made in accordance with the requirements of section 403(r) is not a drug solely because the label or the labeling contains such a claim. A food, dietary ingredient, or dietary supplement for which a truthful and not misleading statement is made in accordance with section 403(r)(6) is not a drug under clause (C) solely because the label or the labeling contains such a statement.

The manner in which the FDA is enforcing this portion of the law, i.e., actually treating dietary supplements like drugs and disallowing supplement claims of almost any kind, is no more than a patently obvious device to enshrine prescription drugs in a preeminent place above every other means of health care treatment. The lengths to which Big Pharma has gone to protect that preeminence, some of which have been presented in this book, are prima facie evidence that this is nothing more than a courtesy which the FDA has bestowed upon its 'clients' in the pharmaceutical industry to protect their collective profitability, at the expense of both the natural products industry and the collective health of the American public.

In contrast, there is a large body of knowledge, gathered from across the planet and across many millenia, that proves that any substance ingested or absorbed by the human body exerts some degree of pharmaceutical effect. If we follow the logic of the FDA's definitions, and the medical/pharmaceutical/insurance complex's employment of them, to its conclusion, are we really going to classify everything we eat, drink or put on our skin as a drug? Don't be absurd! Rather, a drug should be defined as any *synthetic* article that exerts such an effect.

Additionally, the Act needs to incorporate the majority of Rep. Ron Paul's (R-TX) HRs 2044 and 2045, filed during the 112th Congress, which allow qualified health claims for natural products, and constrain the ability of the FDA's partner in crime, the Federal Trade Commission, from unfairly harassing the natural products industry. Congressman Paul has long been a stalwart defender of our health freedom.

If we're serious about containing health care costs, we need to adopt an 'outcome based' mentality, rather than an 'evidence based' one. What is the difference between the two?

In 'evidenced based' research, the focus and emphasis is primarily on the methodology being employed to obtain the result. As mentioned earlier, this can give rise to truly meaningless results, such as "*the operation was a success, but the patient died.*" By enshrining the methodology over the attainment of meaningful results, the importance of the effect on the patient fades into the background, ultimately giving rise to the mindset characterized by the quote above.

In contrast, the 'outcome based' paradigm focuses on a sole criterion: did the remedy or therapy work? In other words, does the patient feel better? Is the health complaint resolved or alleviated? Here, the focus is primarily on the patient, not the methodology. If the remedy/therapy is safe, if it works, if it is cost effective, and can be easily and cheaply offered to large numbers of people, it should be made widely available to the public.

Also, the FDA Reform Act should mandate that the authors of any research that the FDA uses to make or approve a health claim disclose all their financial ties with any food or drug company. When a research study is cited by a governmental regulatory body to determine the safety and/or effectiveness of a certain food, drug or nutritional product, the sponsorship and funding source for that study must be disclosed and evaluated as a factor in determining the accuracy of the research. Failure to do so should carry substantial criminal and financial penalties, for both FDA officials who ignore the requirement as well as researchers who do so.

If the FDA is unable to determine that financial information, it should be required to treat that information as inherently suspect and not use it or refer to it as part of the approval process. If the study is commissioned by a non-profit organization or think tank (a favorite mechanism of businesses to conceal their involvement in a research project), the organizations or companies funding that non-profit organization, as well as the level of funding, must be disclosed.

Finally, the FDA should be required to accept as valid both historical and empirical information about the safety and effectiveness of non-drug and non-surgical therapies. As was demonstrated earlier, the placebo controlled, clinical double blind study has inherent weaknesses that leave it open to exploitation for financial gain. At the same time, the vast data base on natural and alternative therapies literally stretches across the planet and spans millennia of time. The American public has a right to access the full extent of this information, unfiltered by institutional bias or financial interest.

Recommendation #4: Demand More Accountability in Health Reporting From the Media. Use the persuasive powers of the executive branch public information system to sensitize the media to the importance of reporting on the financial aspects of health care research, to include emphasis on potential conflicts of interest in the reporting of health care-related studies.

Here is where the 'bully pulpit' of the executive branch of the federal government could exert great, positive influence upon the news media to clean up their act in the area of health reporting. Actually, all it would take is one major newspaper, TV network or magazine to drop their slavish dependence upon drug advertising, and embark on an independent inquiry, for the rest of the industry to follow suit.

Why would it be that easy? Everyone in the media loves the 'scoop,' the story that trumps everyone else in the profession. As you've seen from just the few stories I've related in this book, there's plenty of ammunition to provide hungry reporters numerous scoops. Once the process begins, we'll be well on our way toward truly reforming our health care system, as opposed to just tinkering around the edges, in deference to the media's financiers.

Recommendation #5: Reform the health insurance industry. Since the industry is governed primarily at the state level, it will require the action of a few bold state governors to set the wheels of this effort in motion. As a first step, state insurance boards could require reimbursement of a wider spectrum of both natural and alternative health care therapies by insurance companies doing business in their state.

As the study I previously cited clearly demonstrated, natural and alternative health care practitioners as primary care providers would save each state an enormous amount of money, and improve health outcomes for millions of citizens. The states could also offer incentives for companies doing business in their state to purchase insurance programs which offer substantial preventive components. Structuring programs around a combination of fitness training, wellness counseling by CAM practitioners, and partnerships between insurance providers and natural products companies holds the promise of measurable, positive increases in health outcomes for millions of people. If individual citizens demand this from their employers and elected officials, our chances of a bright, healthful individual and societal future are materially increased.

Additionally, the Secretary of Health and Human Services should convene a committee to identify opportunities for incorporating more complementary and alternative health care services into existing health care insurance plans. The committee could make recommendations to the Secretary on how to work with the insurance industry to best incorporate those modalities that hold the most promise for reducing consumer costs.

Recommendation #6: Provide incentives for farmers to more strategically employ farmland and fully fertilize their crops so that the nutrient shortfalls previously identified are closed. This would go a long way toward closing the nutritional gap, by not only improving dietary nutrient values but also reducing healthcare costs as a result of improving Americans' diets. The President should convene a Department of Agriculture commission to create a set of tasks to accomplish this goal, and provide the Secretary of Agriculture a report, with recommendations on how to implement them.

Recommendation #7: Create incentives for cities and states to make complementary and alternative health care services more visible, accessible and affordable to the average citizen, thus helping to reduce the city and state health care cost burden. As the previously cited studies clearly demonstrate, properly employed CAM can help facilitate huge reductions in health care costs. This initiative may include, but not be limited to, making federal funding assistance for state health care programs contingent upon the passage of 'safe harbor' and/or title legislation to increase the visibility and accessibility of complementary and alternative practitioners, and rescinding of state laws which limit current access and drive up costs.

The term 'safe harbor' means that an unlicensed complementary and alternative health care practitioner is exempt from the provisions of a given state's medical practice act, provided that the practitioner does not engage in activity specifically prohibited by that state's government, and fully discloses their professional training, qualifications and theory of practice to the consumer. This type of law has been successfully enacted in eight states, greatly expanding the visibility and availability of CAM services in those states, and protecting practitioners from unwarranted prosecution for technical violations of the too-broad provisions of the medical practice act.

In contrast, a title act spells out the requirements practitioners must meet in order to legally claim the use of a specific title. For example, while there are many types of nutritionists practicing in the US, the title "*certified clinical nutritionist*," or CCN, is reserved for those who have completed very specific types of clinically oriented nutritional education and training. The advantage of this type of legislation is that it helps clarify for the consumer exactly what the qualifications of the practitioner are, without having to establish the expensive, cumbersome state-managed infrastructure associated with a full blown licensing law.

Examples of restrictive licensing laws which act as impediments to greater consumer access include:

- Exclusionary licensing laws, such as those pursued by the Academy of Nutrition and Dietetics, that confer sole ownership of a field of complementary and alternative health care to a single community;
- Laws which prohibit or restrict currently licensed health care professionals from practicing complementary and alternative medicine;
- Laws which bar complementary and alternative health care professions from meaningful participation in state health care policy decisions.

Recommendation #8: Better synchronize the actions of US public health care officials in the international arena with the overall objectives of our reformed health care system. This will require FDA officials who represent the United States to use the altered definitions of foods and drugs in Recommendation #3 above as a national position in the ongoing CODEX negotiations, mentioned in Chapter 7. They should also be barred from advocating for 'normalization' of food and dietary supplement values, and allow the US natural products industry to continue to adhere to the guidance offered in the 1994 Dietary Supplement Health and Education Act (DSHEA).

Recommendation #9: Develop a national strategy for dealing with toxic exposure in our society. Create a task force, composed of leading experts in the complementary and alternative health care, environmental quality, occupational health and safety, and labor communities to craft a comprehensive strategy for dealing with the chemical, biological, radiological and electronic threats to public health. The strategy should include identification of specific threats, identification of professional communities and resources best suited to counter the threats, and creation of a public education strategy to bring the threats and resources to the American public's attention. Responsibility for implementation should be divided among the appropriate executive branch agencies. The task force should present its report to the Secretaries of Health and Human Services and Labor, and the Director of the Environmental Protection Agency, for immediate implementation.

Recommendation #10: Develop a national strategy for effective stress management in our society, providing both improved health and reduced healthcare costs. Convene a panel of experts, with substantial emphasis on the field of complementary and alternative health care, to create a set of guidelines and develop a comprehensive strategy for managing all aspects of the major categories of stress in our society. The panel should also include expertise from the arenas of public health, environmental health and quality, and labor, to provide maximum cross-disciplinary input for creating usable solutions. The panel will present its results to the Secretaries of Health and Human Services and Labor, and the Director of the Environmental Protection Agency, with recommendations for immediate implementation.

How You Can Help. Obviously, these recommendations will only be enacted with substantial input and demand from our fellow citizens. In a democratic republic, the ultimate power to govern is supposed to rest with the people. As you have seen throughout this book, segments of the health care system have, for reasons of their own, gradually eroded the ability of the US people to manage their most important asset: their health. Those same segments continue to do so because they collectively do not think our fellow citizens are sufficiently well educated to make those decisions, so someone has to make the decisions for them, and because they believe our fellow citizens do not possess the strength of will to act decisively in their own interests. This is in direct conflict with the guidance Thomas Jefferson offered us so long ago:

"I know of no safe depository of the ultimate powers of the society but the people themselves, and if we think them not enlightened enough to exercise control with a wholesome discretion, the remedy is not to take it from them, but to inform their discretion by education." (*Thomas Jefferson, letter to William C. Jarvis, September 28, 1820*)

Unfortunately, when this kind of power is bestowed wholesale upon a single community without adequate checks and balances, it opens the door for abuse of that power. We have seen that the desire for monetary gain, disguised as the desire to 'protect the public,' has created a health care oligarchy that wields immense power to serve its own ends, to the point where it is creating immense economic, political and health dislocation in our society.

But what to do about it? As I mentioned in the Preface, *Adrenaline Nation* is part of a campaign to bring to the American people's attention the scale of the problem of chronic stress in our society, and to propose meaningful solutions to that problem. Inextricably bound to that campaign is another: to alert the American people to the direct threat that the current health care system poses to our individual freedom to choose. Both of these goals are wholeheartedly supported by both my publisher, Smart Publications, and the dedicated network of thousands of health freedom advocates around the country and the globe who, unbeknownst to most people, strive daily to protect *your* freedom to choose.

Smart Publications has dedicated a set of pages on their web site to these causes, which has both links to important health freedom information, including currently filed legislation, and sample letters that you can adapt to contact your elected representatives and make your voice heard. Please go to the main page for this book

-- www.smart-publications/books/adrenaline-nation/ -- and click on the 'Health Freedom' link. We invite you to join us in making a difference to improve our collective physical and fiscal health, that of our children, and most of all, to protect the hard won freedoms we all so dearly cherish.

"It's Not Nice to Fool With Mother Nature." As we've seen clearly in this book, despite all the benefits and advancements of contemporary society and medical science, it is dangerous to subscribe to the intellectual arrogance, as we often have done, that modern man has surpassed Mother Nature's level of sophistication, comprehensiveness and effectiveness.

From our earliest days on this planet, man woke and slept according to the rising and the setting of the sun, ate fresh food that was hunted or gathered, exerted physical effort to ensure his survival, looked to nature's garden for healing, and to the natural process for guidance. The more advanced our society has become, the more disconnected we have become from both this timeless collective wisdom and the ever present signals from our bodies which provide the ultimate source of truth.

The importance of adhering to this natural guidance was emphasized very clearly in the previously mentioned quote by Sir Ken Robinson, PhD, from his best-selling book *The Element*. Now is the time for us, as individuals and as a society, to reconnect with that timeless source of wisdom and health that exists within each of us. It's been there all along, waiting for us to notice it and re-engage with it. The most effective means of accelerating our journey along that path is to strike the correct balance between man's ingenuity and Nature's power, majesty and innate wisdom.

As Thomas Edison stated so long ago, we are on the threshold of immense advances in virtually every field of human endeavor. We are so fortunate to be living at a time in human history when "*we are now, a-tremble on the verge of vast discoveries - discoveries so wondrously important they will upset the present trend of human thought and start it along completely new lines."*

Let us not retreat in fear from this opportunity and misguidedly cling to outdated self-interest; rather, let us face that future with boldness, compassion for our fellow men, respect and admiration for the Universe which is our cradle and home, and the wisdom to use all our available tools to fashion a future our children will be proud of.

Resource Listing

For your convenience, I have organized the resources referenced throughout the book by chapter. If the resource is referenced more than once, it is placed in the chapter where it is first referred to. Also, since the body of health knowledge is expanding so rapidly, please check the Smart Publications website at www.smart-publications.com/books/adrenaline-nation/ frequently for the most up-to-date resource information.

Preface

Chopra, Deepak, *Creating Affluence: The A-to-Z Steps to a Richer Life*, Amber-Allen Publishing, San Rafael, CA, 1998.

Chapter 1

Mosby's Medical Encyclopedia, The Complete Home Medical Reference, Software by Broderbund, available through www.Amazon.com.

The Free Dictionary - www.thefreedictionary.com

Wikipedia - www.wikipedia.org

The American Institute of Stress - www.stress.org

MedicineNet – www.MedicineNet.com

Time Thoughts – www.TimeThoughts.com

Cherniski, Stephen, *Caffeine Blues: Wake Up to the Hidden Dangers of America's #1 Drug*, Warner Books, Inc., New York, NY, 1998.

Batmanghelidj, Fereydoon MD, *Your Body's Many Cries for Water*, Global Health Solutions, Inc., Vienna, VA, 1997.

Gerber, Richard MD, *Vibrational Medicine for the 21st Century*, William Morrow/HarperCollins Publishers, New York, NY, 2000.

Chaitow, Leon, DO, *Fibromyalgia Syndrome: A Practitioner's Guide to Treatment*, Churchill Livingstone, New York, NY, 2003.

Goodwin, James S. MD and Tangum, Michael R. MD, *Battling Quackery: Attitudes About Micronutrient Supplements in American Academic Medicine*, ARCH INTERN MED/Vol. 158, Nov. 9, 1998, pgs. 2187-2191.

Davis, D. PhD, FACN, Epp, M. PhD and Riordan, H. MD, *Changes in USDA Food Composition Data for 43 Garden Crops, 1950 to 1999*, Journal of the American College of Nutrition, Vol. 23, No. 6, 669–682 (2004).

Fitzgerald, Patricia, *The Detox Solution: The Missing Link to Radiant Health, Abundant Energy, Ideal Weight and Peace of Mind*, Illumination Press, Santa Monica, CA, 2001.

Chapter 2

Dyer, Wayne PhD, *Excuses Begone! How to Change Lifelong, Self-Defeating Thinking Habits*, Hay House, Inc., Carlsbad, CA, 2009.

Miller, Lyle H. PhD, and Smith, Alma Dell PhD, *The Stress Solution: An Action Plan to Manage the Stress In Your Life*, Pocket Books, New York, NY, 1993.

American Psychological Association (APA) - www.apa.org

Johnson, Spencer, *Who Moved My Cheese?: An Amazing Way to Deal with Change in Your Work and in Your Life*, Penguin Putnam, Inc., New York, NY, 2002.

Chapter 3

Philip S. Wang, M.D., Dr.P.H., Arne L. Beck, Ph.D., Pat Berglund, M.B.A., David K. McKenas, M.D., M.P.H., Nicolaas P. Pronk, Ph.D., Gregory E. Simon, M.D., M.P.H., Ronald C. Kessler, Ph.D., *Effects of Major Depression on Moment-in-Time Work Performance*, American Journal of Psychiatry 2004; 161:1885–1891.

Carlo, Dr. George PhD, and Schramm, Martin, *Cell Phones: Invisible Hazards in the Wireless Age*, Carroll & Graf Publishers, New York, NY, 2001.

Schlosser, Eric, *Fast Food Nation: The Dark Side of the All-American Meal*, HarperCollins Publishers, New York, NY, 2003.

Khurana, Vini Gautam, PhD, FRACS, *Mobile Phones and Brain Tumours – A Public Health Concern*, 2008. Available online.

Kirn, Walter, *The Autumn of the Multitaskers*, The Atlantic, November 2007.

Chapter 4

Muller, Rev. Wayne, *Sabbath: Finding Rest, Renewal, and Delight in Our Busy Lives*, Bantam Books/Random House, Inc., New York, NY, 1999.

Sapolsky, Robert M., *Why Zebras Don't Get Ulcers: An Updated Guide to Stress, Stress Related Diseases, and Coping (2nd Edition)*, W. H. Freeman, New York, NY, 1998.

Pearce, Joseph Chilton, *The Biology of Transcendence: A Blueprint of the Human Spirit*, Park Street Press, Rochester, VT, 2004.

Chapter 7

Prochaska J.O., Velicer W.F. *The Transtheoretical Model of Health Behavior Change*, Am J Health Promot., 1997 Sep-Oct;12(1):38-48.

CODEX Articles by Peter Byrne:
www.smart-publications.com/articles/the-codex-agenda-and-what-it-means-for-dietary-supplements/
www.smart-publications.com/articles/the-history-of-codex-and-the-fate-of-vitamins/

Chapter 8

Whole Foods' Health Care reform article: http://online.wsj.com/article/SB10001424052970204251404574342170072865070.html

National Center for Complementary and Alternative Medicine (NCCAM: http://nccam.nih.gov/)

Smith, Alan, *UnBreak Your Health*, Loving Healing Press, Ann Arbor, MI, 2010. www.unbreakyourhealth.com/

Smart Publications Health and Wellness E-newsletter: www.smart-publications.com/subscribe/

Longevity Medicine Review: www.lmreview.com/

Jonathan Wright, MD: http://wrightnewsletter.com/

Garry Gordon, DO, MD: www.longevityplus.com/

Marianne Marchese, ND: www.townsendletter.com/search.htm
To find Dr. Marchese's specific articles, use the following link:
http://townsendletter.master.com/texis/master/search/mysite.html?
q=Marianne+Marchese&submit=Search+this+site

Life Extension Foundation: www.lef.org/

American Botanical Council: http://abc.herbalgram.org/

Elaine Masters' Drivetime Yoga/Flytime Yoga: www.drivetimeyoga.
com/

Wolever, Thomas MD, PhD, and Brand-Miller, Jennie PhD et al,
*The Glucose Revolution: The Authoritative Guide to the Glycemic
Index*, Marlowe & Company, New York, NY, 1999.

D'Adamo, Dr. Peter J., *Eat Right 4 Your Type*, Riverhead Books,
New York, NY, 2002.

John A. Amaro, DC, FIAMA, Dipl. Ac., L.Ac.: www.iama.edu/
JetLag/JetLag.htm

Bach Flower Remedies – how to find a practitioner
www.bachcentre.com/found/rp_ref.htm

Eker, T. Harv, *Secrets of the Millionaire Mind*, HarperBusiness,
Harper Collins Publishers, New York, NY, 2005.

Meditation Resources:
Brantley, Jeffrey, MD, *Calming Your Anxious Mind*, New Harbinger Publications, Inc., Oakland, CA, 2003.

A wide variety of meditation resources (books, tapes, and DVDs) sponsored and endorsed by Deepak Chopra, MD are available at Wild Divine: www.wilddivine.com/

Hanh, Thich Nhat, *The Miracle of Mindfulness: An Introduction to the Practice of Meditation*, Beacon Press, Boston, MA, 1976.

Creative Visualization and Relaxation (CVR): www.newreality.com

Health Freedom Nutrition: www.hfn-usa.com

Health Care Practitioners:
IMPORTANT NOTE: The organizations listed below are offered strictly as an easy means of locating practitioners who are members of the respective organizations. There are many others who don't belong to these organizations and are equally capable. Please check locally as well.

Homeopathy:
www.homeopathic.org/resources/practitioners

www.homeopathy.org/directory_entrance.html

Asian Medicine:
As you will discover, there are a large number of reputable Asian medicine schools and practitioners. Their availability varies from state to state. To find an Asian medicine practitioner in your area, Google Asian medicine AND (your home state).

Chiropractic:
www.acatoday.org/search/memsearch.cfm

Rolfing:
www.rolf.org/find

Massage:
www.amtamassage.org/findamassage /index.html

American Holistic Medical Association:
www.holisticmedicine.org/AF_MemberDirectory.asp

American Association of Naturopathic Physicians:
www.naturopathic.org/AF_MemberDirectory.asp?version=1

American Naturopathic Medical Association:
150 South Highway 160, Ste. 8-528, Pahrump, Nevada 89048, Telephone (888) 202-4440 Fax (888) 502-3385. Call for practitioner information.

International and American Association of Clinical Nutritionists:
www.iaacn.org/contactpage.htm

Ayurvedic Medicine:
Like Asian medicine, there are a large number of reputable Ayurveidc medicine schools and practitioners. Their availability varies from state to state. To find an Ayurvedic medicine practitioner in your area, Google Ayurvedic medicine AND (your home state).

Apex Energetics:
If you are not a licensed practitioner, you can email a request to info@apexenergetics.com, and they can find a practitioner in your area for you who uses their training and products.

Energetix:
www.goenergetix.com/find-a-practitioner

Ober, Clinton, Sinatra, Stephen, MD, and Zucker, Martin, *Earthing: The Most Important Health Discovery Ever?*, Basic Health Publications, Inc., Laguna Beach, CA, 2010.

GIA/BioPro:
www.cellphone-health.com/

Waiora Natural Cellular Defense: www.waiora.com/products/pro_ncd.p

REFERENCES

[i] MacLennan AH, Wilson DH, Taylor AW: The escalating cost and prevalence of alternative medicine. Preventive Medicine 2002, 35:166-173.

[ii] DaVanzo, J. PhD, MSW, Freeman, J. MA, Effect of Selected Dietary Supplements on Health Care Reduction – Study Update, The Lewin Group, June 5, 2007

[iii] Sarnat, R. MD, Winterstein, J. DC, Cambron, J. DC, PhD. Clinical Utilization and Cost Outcomes From an Integrative Medicine Independent Physician Association: An Additional 3-Year Update, Journal of Manipulative and Physiological Therapeutics, May 2007, pgs. 263-269.

[iv]Ibid., pg. 263.

[v] White AR, Resch KL, Ernst E, Methods of economic evaluation in complementary medicine. Forsch Komplementarmed 1996, 3:196-203.

[vi] www.photius.com/rankings/world_health_performance_ranks.html

[vii] Sarnat, Winterstein, et al, pgs. 263-269.

[viii] www.forbes.com/2005/02/24/cx_mh_0224fda.html

[ix] Faloon, W., Dietary Supplements Attacked by the Media, Life Extension Magazine, June 2006, p. 1.

[x] Ibid. pgs. 1, 2, 4, 9.

[xi] Null, G. PhD, Dean, C. MD ND, Feldman, M. MD, Rasio, D. MD, Smith, D. PhD, Death by Medicine, Life Extension Institute, October 2003.

[xii] Ltr from David L. Lakey, MD, Commissioner Texas Department of State Health Services, to Rep. Patrick Rose, October 24, 2007, p. 2.

[xiii] www.eatright.org/corporatesponsors

INDEX

H

I